I'M NOT CRAZY

(I'M JUST A TAD DITZY)

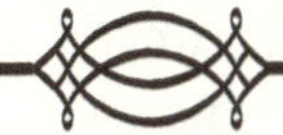

AN ODYSSEY TO DIAGNOSIS OF RELAPSING-REMITTING MULTIPLE SCLEROSIS

Jeanne Phaneuf Champagne

ISBN 978-1-64300-372-6 (Paperback)
ISBN 978-1-64300-373-3 (Digital)

Covenant Books, Inc.
11661 Hwy 707
Murrells Inlet, SC 29576
www.covenantbooks.com

DEDICATION

I am incredibly blessed to share my life with a cherished companion who has partnered with me through thick and thin since the day we met. No one has loved me more deeply, more consistently, or more sacrificially than this easygoing, kind-hearted man. His positive view of life has tremendously influenced my own outlook and fueled me with optimism. Even when circumstances are sometimes not very funny, he has a unique way of bringing out the laughter in me. I am deeply grateful to God for this man. If there is anything worth dedicating through these pages, I humbly dedicate this work to Dennis Champagne, my beloved husband and life-long soul mate since 1971.

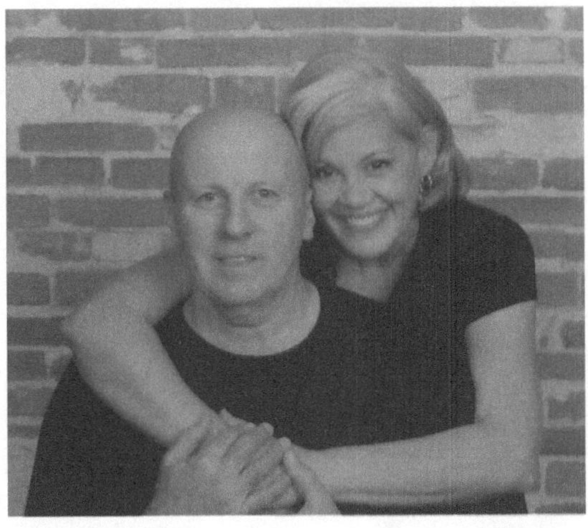

CHAPTER ONE

A BOOK? REALLY? WHY WRITE A BOOK?

Every human alive has a story. Mine may not be exceptional to some, but it is *my* story. This book is about just one chapter in this life—my personal journey with relapsing-remitting multiple sclerosis (RRMS).

Initially, writing was my awkward attempt at telling those I love how I was personally, emotionally, physiologically, cognitively, and socially affected by MS. Although I recognized that multiple sclerosis is not a death sentence, for nearly fifteen years, I had no idea that the broad spectrum of symptoms that infiltrated my life was interrelated. Doctors and specialists didn't put two-plus-two together, and for reasons explained later in this book, it is understandable.

To make sense of health issues that started in 1997, I managed to retain records from which the details of this book were written. It wasn't until 2013 that neurological tests and an MRI revealed that these collective symptoms had a name. I was diagnosed with multiple sclerosis—more specifically, *relapsing-remitting multiple sclerosis.*

I had known for a *long* time that *something* was amiss, so it wasn't a big deal accepting the diagnosis of MS. My personal challenge was accepting the losses that accompanied "whatever it was." Admittedly, there were times I felt a teensy bit sorry for myself as favorite activities like ballroom dancing, playing guitar, or taking a brisk walk became more challenging. Like anyone who loses the ability to do things we love, I had moments when I mourned the loss of these old "friends."

My experience of a long, drawn-out diagnosis is common among those with this perplexing and often ambiguous disease. I found that learning all I could about MS empowered me to deal more effectively with its unpredictable and haphazard symptoms and concluded that if I found it challenging to deal with issues ignited by MS, then others must too. If my experiences could help others navigate their way more smoothly through the complex maze of MS, I felt compelled to share them.

As my fingers began flying across the keyboard in an effort to write my story, I discovered how difficult it was to be truly open about my journey and the countless symptoms I'd habitually covered for *so* long. I needed to share it if for no one else's sake but my own. My struggles were showing, and it was becoming more difficult to hide them than it was to live with them openly. I knew the jig was up. Hiding was no longer an option.

That's when the writing of this book began.

CHAPTER TWO

THE FLU THAT IGNITED THE TORCH

My personal journey with relapsing-remitting multiple sclerosis began in February of 1997. Of course, I didn't know I had MS at the time. In fact, it would be nearly fifteen years before I learned what was plaguing me. Not dealing with life-threatening issues, I pretty much just coasted along. Yet in my own mind, there was a clear and definite marker when my brain went "haywire" and an aspect of my life changed from that point forward.

The Flu

Dennis had a long-planned mission trip to Panama to which he had been looking forward for months. Several weeks before his departure, we both caught an acute upper respiratory virus (i.e. the "flu.") We were so sick with fever, chills, headache, and fatigue, we were barely able to care for ourselves, much less for one another! By the end of the third week, Dennis was feeling much better, but my body was still taking its jolly old time getting well.

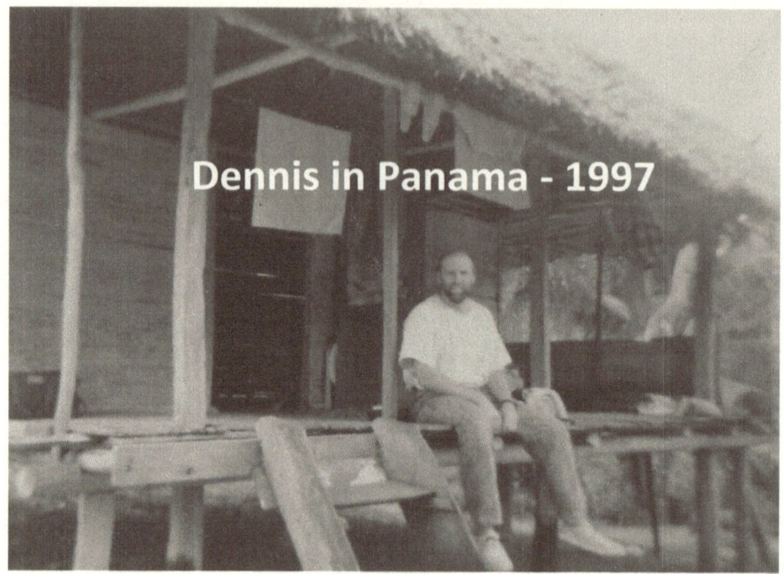

The day of Dennis's departure arrived, and off he flew to Panama where he would be unreachable for over a month. I had to convince him to go, as he felt badly leaving me still feeling so puny. I was sure I'd start feeling better soon, and a week or so later, I felt well enough to get out of bed for longer periods of time.

I wasn't up more than a few days when my friend Sally invited me to join her for a trip to the grocery store. Though I wasn't fully recovered, I did need groceries, so I agreed to accompany her. Once there, we went our separate ways arranging to meet at the front of the store. We weren't there long before I started feeling lightheaded and weak. I pushed forward, trying to ignore how I felt, but by the time I reached the back of the store, I was *utterly* disoriented. I could hear the inside of my head pounding in my ears and thought, "I need to find Sally!"

My next recollection was looking upward into a circle of strangers' faces surrounding me as I lay on the tiled floor. I could not move my arms or legs and had *no* idea where I was or what had happened. I stared half-dazed into unfamiliar faces as paramedics asked me questions. I saw their mouths moving but was unable to comprehend what they were saying. Like a movie in slow motion, their words started to make sense, and I realized they were talking to me.

"Are you diabetic?"

"Did you pass out?"

"Do you have any medical conditions?"

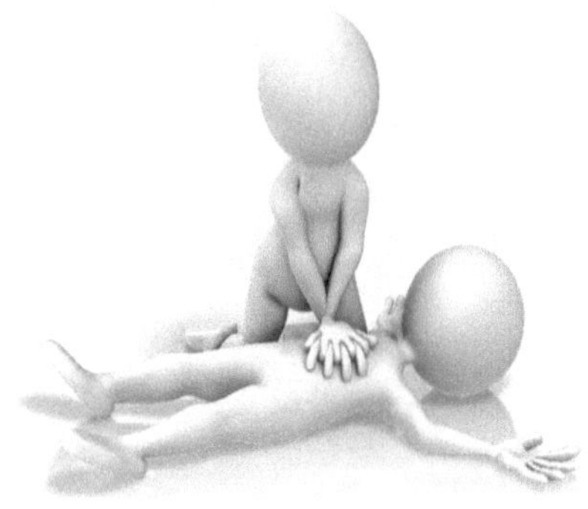

My gaze roamed from face to face before I saw Sally. Recognizing her helped me become more oriented, and I recalled we had traveled together. The paramedics offered to take me by ambulance to the hospital, but I refused transport, informing them that I had been sick and must have gotten out too soon. A few days later, I had another "passing out" episode.

What's Going On?

My memory of the weeks that followed remains a blur as I had *dozens* more loss-of-consciousness episodes. With Dennis still in Panama and unaware of these issues, my brother made the decision on my behalf to take me to the hospital. Only a few isolated, hazy memories of that time flicker through my mind—the faces of people with whom I went to church, someone trying to feed me, a woman's voice saying emphatically, "*This is not good!*" and the voices of different people praying out loud for me. I was so exhausted and "out of it" that, initially, I didn't even realize I was in the hospital.

One night, I was awake enough to realize Dennis was far away and aware enough to comprehend I was lying in a hospital bed, but I had no idea how I got there or why. It was very quiet in the room and halls when suddenly an overwhelming wave of fear washed over me. I felt exceedingly vulnerable—like a bad dream from which I could not awaken.

"Am I sick?" I asked myself as my surroundings became clearer.

"How did I get here … *Why* am I here?"

"Am I dying?" A sense of helplessness overcame me.

"Dear God, *please don't let me die*," I pleaded. I feared that if I died, Dennis wouldn't find out until he returned. "I don't want to disappear out my family's lives," I cried out to God. "They'll be devastated!"

I thought about my own mother "disappearing" out of her seven children's lives. She died of a brain aneurysm following a simple gallbladder surgery. Now, here I was in the hospital possibly having brain issues, and no one knew why! I wept uncontrollably but very quietly in that room. I didn't want the hospital staff to hear me or know just how terrified and confused I was. I never felt so alone.

As I wept, a nurse entered my room, pulled a chair up close, took my hands in hers, and in a voice of incredible compassion, whispered, "Don't worry, sweetie. *Everything is going to be okay.*"

I can't articulate how profoundly comforted I was by this nurse's compassion. With her words came the palpable presence of the Spirit of Comfort that filled the entire room and encompassed me. I have never forgotten that moment, and to this day, I believe wholeheartedly that I was embraced by God Himself through this nurse angel.

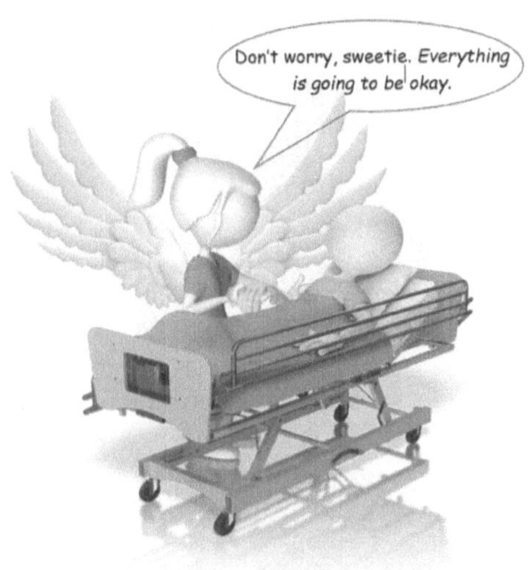

When Dennis and the missionaries returned from Panama's interior, he was informed that I had been hospitalized and took the first available flight home. He'd been away nearly three weeks, and I was quite ready for his return!

The Un-Special "Specialist"

During and after my hospital stay, dangerously elevated blood pressure concerned the doctors. For months following that flu, doctors attempted unsuccessfully to bring it under control. I was referred to a hematologist who ran tests and scans before sending me to a cardiologist who ran his own tests determining that, although I had an irregular heartbeat, there was nothing life-threateningly wrong with my heart. The cardiologist then referred me to an endocrinologist, and it was with this "specialist" that my confidence in doctors was annihilated.

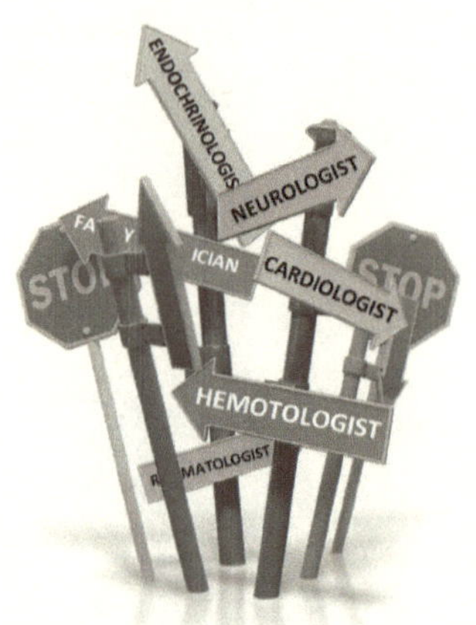

Entering the room with a condescending air, this "specialist" seemed annoyed that a patient occupied his exam room. "Why are you here?" he flatly asked, leaning against the wall with his arms crossed. I was already inexplicably drained from "whatever it was" causing these episodes, but now I felt rushed and intimidated. However, I was there for a purpose, so once again, I told *another* specialist about the flu, the passing out episodes, and anything else I thought was pertinent. I was very aware of the annoyed frown on this doctor's face as he rolled his eyes and sighed out loud as I talked. If I'd have felt better, I would have walked out the door. Instead, I stood there, exhausted, as this insensitive character, who knew me fewer than ten minutes, responded in an arrogant tone, "Maybe what *you* need is a psychiatrist."

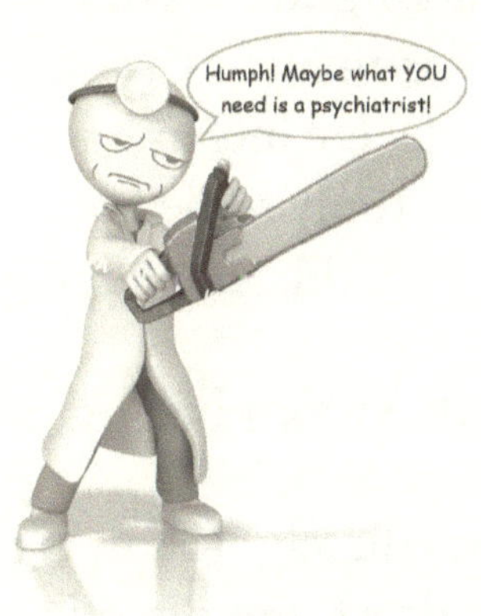

I'm sure my chin dropped to the floor at his comment. I was truly stunned and didn't even know what to say. *This* was his conclusion? His reply did not mesh well with how physically and neurologically "out of sorts" I was, and his response had a long-lasting and negative impact on how I would view doctors for a *very* long time. After this experience and months of no answers, I even began to question myself. *Was this all in my head?*

It would be nearly four months and innumerable "passing out" episodes before I would go back to *anyone* in the medical field. *I was done!* Instead, I dealt with these and a multitude of other symptoms with a helpless sense about what to do. In 1997, access to reputable medical information websites was not so readily available, so figuring things out on one's own was far more challenging in a day when many doctors did not like to be questioned.

As episodes increased, I was relentlessly disoriented and indescribably fatigued. To my dismay, I could not find my way to work and back without being totally *lost*. I had driven that road hundreds of times, but now I could barely find my way out of a parking lot. Dennis chauffeured me back and forth to work. Fortunately, the physical therapists at the clinic where I worked were incredibly patient and knew that when I "disappeared" (only to be found on the floor having another "episode") I would, soon enough, "return."

I Think She's Having Seizures

One day, immediately following another of many "episodes," Dennis drove me directly to a DO (doctor of osteopathic medicine) that one of the physical therapists had recommended. I was still completely disoriented when we arrived. (I recall none of this except that Dennis told me.) The DO performed basic neurological in-office tests, asked me questions, then turned to Dennis and said, "*I think she's having seizures.*" She referred me to a neurologist who ordered a sleep-deprived EEG, which confirmed that the "episodes" I'd been experiencing for nearly five months were right frontal focus "complex partial seizures."

At my follow-up appointment, the neurologist handed me a pamphlet entitled "*Living with Epilepsy.*" I looked at him bewildered and wondered why he just placed *this* pamphlet in my lap.

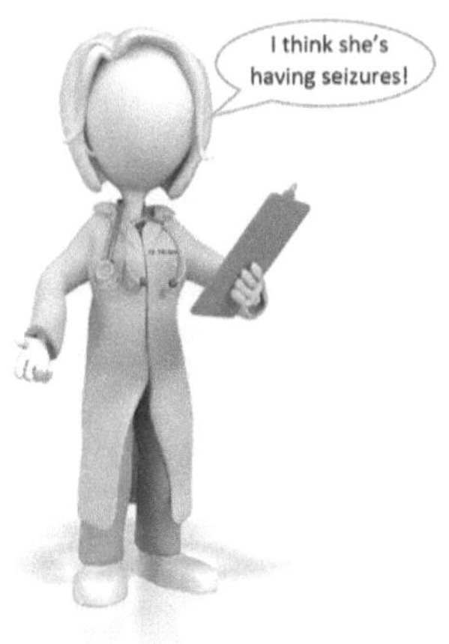

"What is this?" I asked.

"You have epilepsy," he replied without emotion. "Read this pamphlet."

That's pretty much it. After that I heard, "blah blah blah … anticonvulsants … blah blah blah … *for the rest of your life.*"

"*The rest of my LIFE?*" I exclaimed. "WHY? *I only had the flu!*"

He informed me that uncontrolled seizures could lead to worsened seizures … brain damage … etc.

"I simply don't buy that. How can you predict something that far down the road? How can I be on something 'for the rest of my life'? How do we know these seizures won't stop as spontaneously as they started? Why '*the rest of my life*'? Why not five years, or three years?" I demanded to know as I argued my case.

The neurologist patiently listened to my rant until I was ranted out. His expression revealed nothing. He said nothing. He just sat there, looking at me, listening.

"I'll try it for a while and see how I do," I ceded. "But I want to get off them as soon as possible."

CHAMPAGNE, JEANNE D

EEG #: 97-284

This EEG was performed on a 42-year-old female with a histor— —f disorientation, palpitations, visual obs——————
sleep deprived and ——

CHAMPAGNE, JEANNE D 97-176

Jeanne returns. Her EEG is abnormal. She has right frontal focus. I'll go ahead and do an MR of the brain. I have recommended anticonvulsants. She is very reluctant to take those. She has read the pamphlets on epilepsy and has some denial about her illness. Her brother-in-law is a pharmacist. She would like to talk to him and I'll go ahead and see her back after her MR scan. She is having at least two partial seizures per day. I explained the risks, especially having a convulsion. She understands that and the driving issues

CHAMPAGNE, JEANNE D
97-1606

Jeanne comes in today. She has had a number of seizures over the weekend. She has an abnormal EEG. I'll go ahead and start her on Tegretol. I have given her a dosing schedule. I went over the side effects with her. She'll stop if she has a rash or cut the dose in half if she has side effects. I'll plan to see her back in three weeks in follow up.

IMPRESSION: Complex partial seizures

RECEIVED 6/6/97

D ——————————————————————————— ——ysm of frontal theta a— —————————— —he correct electrode placement, appear to ———— ——ght frontal predominance, raising the possibility of focal cerebral dysfunction in that region.

This whole life-long medication thing was a lot to take in, and I was in no frame of mind to be making decisions. I went to my car and did the only thing I knew to do in this situation … I sobbed. It wasn't the diagnosis of epilepsy that hit me like a bolt of lightning, but the idea of taking anticonvulsants *"for the rest of my life."* No pun intended, but that was a lot to swallow!

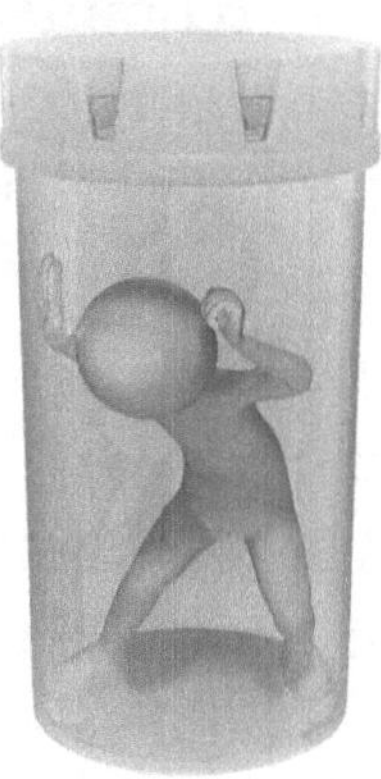

Later, I read my medical report and had to chuckle at the neurologist's comment that I had "some denial about her illness …" *Some* denial? Honestly, you could have knocked me over with the smallest puff of air! Like a defeated puppy, I returned home, fearful about consuming these medications but even more afraid of uncontrolled seizures. Reluctantly, I started the anticonvulsants with the goal in mind to get off them as soon as I could figure out an alternative.

Even on medications, I was still having seizures, so five months later, I visited the Mayo Clinic in Minnesota. A "well-oiled machine," the Mayo Clinic ordered a host of diagnostic testing. The EEG confirmed a seizure disorder, and highly elevated blood pressure continued to be a health concern. Unfortunately, several more days of testing and evaluations offered no definitive diagnosis. The neurology team at Mayo was kind, understanding, and encouraging. They explained that identifying the cause of seizures or maladies of the brain and central nervous system can be challenging if images and tests do not reveal something obvious. "For now," their recommendation was to manage symptoms (seizures and elevated blood pressure) and take on the "wait and see" approach. To keep seizures at bay, the anticonvulsant dosage was increased (much to my dismay), and a new blood pressure lowering medication was added.

Even though I left the Mayo Clinic with more prescriptions than I came (and still without answers), I remained optimistic that my journey there would somehow have a magical outcome, and I would start getting better.

That didn't happen.

CHAPTER THREE

PUZZLE PIECES

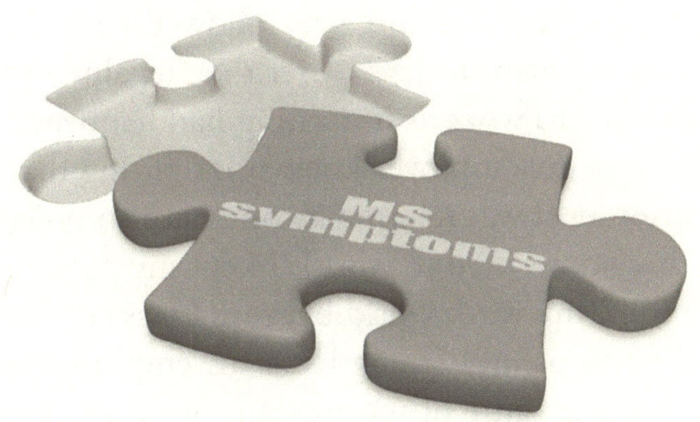

There were many symptoms I never mentioned to doctors as time passed. Somewhat "scarred" by the response of that "specialist" earlier in my quest for answers, I was often hesitant to discuss many of the symptoms that came and went without reason. I didn't want doctors to think I was making it up! While I didn't know what was going on, I *did* know I had been dealing with *something* for a *very* long time and continued to tell doctors for fifteen years that I was certain "that flu" was the beginning of these issues.

Understandably, each doctor treated only the symptom(s) manifesting at the time.

Moving On

Eventually, the physical therapy clinic where I worked was bought out, and I accepted a position as administrator of a multi-location, multi-doctor oral surgery practice. I lost count how many seizures I had behind locked doors on the bathroom floor in my new workplace. Because I could sense when a seizure was coming on, I would make my way to a private area and place myself on the floor. Each complex partial seizure was followed with the inability to move my arms or legs. After they regained function, I would return to work as if nothing had happened.

Although my employer knew upon hiring that I had a seizure disorder (I was referred by one of the physical therapists with whom I used to work), I kept my personal world separate from my work world because I was confident that my qualifications and strengths as an employee were not compromised because of seizures, nor were any shortcomings caused by it. Having seizures and hiding them went on for half a decade with only a few co-workers occasionally informed *only* because, at times, I felt *so* awful I thought someone else should know.

Things That Go "POP"

A few years following the onset of the flu and subsequent seizures and symptoms that ensued, my father became very ill. I flew "back home" to Rhode Island to be with my six siblings and to spend our final days with him. While there, I experienced a painful area in my left calf that nagged and distracted me almost constantly. I tried to ignore it, but the pain grew greater by the day. I was soon to learn that it was two bulged discs in my lumbar spine causing this radiating nerve pain.

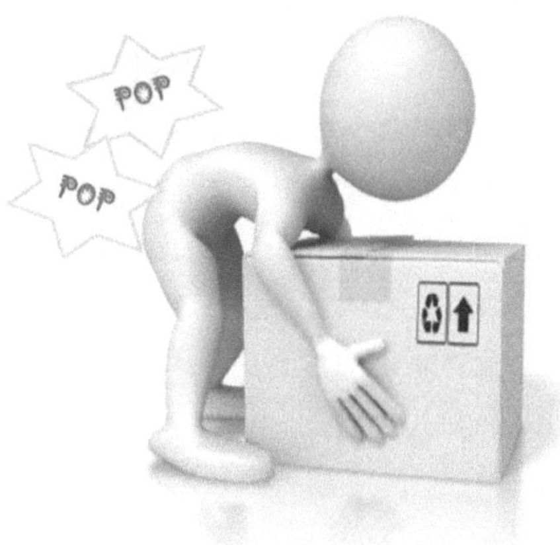

After Dad passed away, I flew back to Arkansas and returned to work, but within a few days, while lifting a heavy box, I felt an odd "pop, pop" in my lower back followed by a hot, flowing sensation. I remember saying to my co-worker, "Uh-oh ... *something bad* just happened!" It was the end of the work week, so I called Dennis, then made my way immediately to my car for the forty-minute drive home. With every passing minute, the pain in my lower back and down my left leg became more excruciating. About ten minutes from home, I was literally screaming in agony and praying out loud, "Dear God, please help me!"

Dennis was outside when I pulled into the driveway. "Honey, I really did it this time!" I cried. "Something snapped in my back while lifting a case of copy paper!" The pain was so unbearable I couldn't budge. Any movement sent searing pain through my back and leg. "Just pull me out," I pleaded in desperation. He wrapped his arms around me in a bear hug and pulled me from the driver's seat. I clung to Dennis, frozen in pain.

"Let's get you in the house," he urged while doing his best to help me up the stairs. I moaned in anguish with every step. Finally, inside the house, we both realized I needed to go to the ER! I couldn't sit, stand, or lie down. There was no relief or position to ease the pain. With no small effort, we made our way back to the car, and I groaned like a distressed animal all the way to the ER where my neurologist met us. With one quick lift of my leg (and one tortured scream from my throat) he told Dennis, "She has a ruptured disc. I'll order an MRI."

Because the radiology department misunderstood the neurologist's order and mistakenly took an image of my cervical spine instead of my back, the MRI now involved *two* trips. I was in too much pain to notice, but after all that agony to get me on the MRI table then back off again, they now had to take me for a *second* one—each movement elicited tormenting pain!

The MRI revealed two ruptured discs in my lumbar spine. I was admitted for pain management until the neurosurgeon could see me in the morning at which time he informed me that "80 percent of patients with ruptured discs can heal without surgery if given time." That's pretty good odds, and I was determined to be among that statistic. If time was all that was needed, I would surely win this battle no matter how torturous. Yet here I was, in my early forties, lying helpless on a gurney like a ninety-year-old woman!

Now, to Touch on the Psychological Side …

I'd spent a lifetime in fear of hospitals. I and my siblings bore the scar of losing our mother needlessly and unexpectedly following a routine gallbladder operation. Immediately after surgery and over the next few days, Mom complained of horrible headaches. My father repeatedly told hospital staff that something was terribly wrong and that she was not herself. His concerns for his beloved wife were not taken seriously. Within days, Mom did not recognize my father or her own children. The family doctor was out of town, and there was no follow up on her care. Mom slipped into a coma, and several days later, at age forty-six, she died of a brain aneurysm. In my mind (and in the minds of my six siblings), hospitals became a place where healthy people go to die. *There was no way I was going to have surgery for my back!*

I was ten days in the hospital on a morphine drip for pain management in hopes that the ruptured discs would "repair themselves." Every day was agony even on medication. Unable to move, sit up, turn over, or get out of bed, even placing a bed pan under me was excruciating. On day ten, the neurosurgeon gave me the news I didn't want to hear—I was not one of those "80 percent" that heals with time.

"I'm sorry to tell you this," he said compassionately, "but you *need* surgery."

I knew he was right. The pain was by far the worst I'd ever experienced, yet to me, having surgery was like tossing a coin in the air: heads, I live; tails, I die. There would certainly be no quality of life in this much anguish, so with all reluctance, I was forced to succumb to surgery. I consciously, prayerfully put my life in God's hands, and once again, I was asking Him, "Please, Lord, don't let me die!"

I know my reaction to having surgery seems a bit dramatic, but losing my mother so needlessly had left its scar and affected me and my family deeply. My faith was all I had, and soon I would find that my faith was all I needed.

Those Wonderful Ceiling Tiles!

Before being wheeled away to surgery the next morning, I said goodbye to Dennis and my children. They had no idea how much I was *really* saying goodbye! Imagine the elation I had when, after surgery, I opened my eyes and saw ceiling tiles! My first thought was, *"I made it! I made it! Thank you, Lord, for letting me live!"*

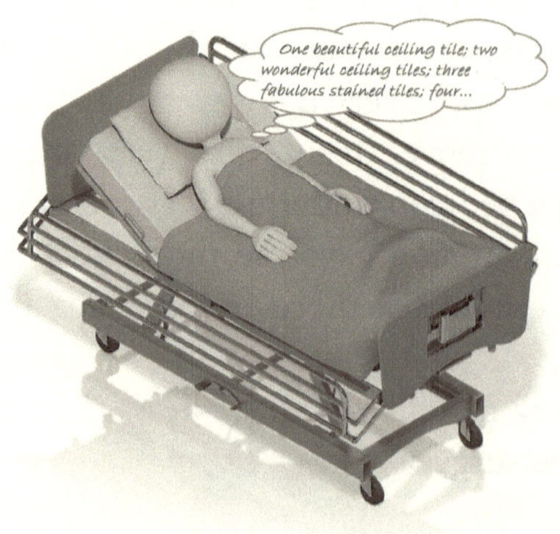

WHEW! Though it wasn't even a "close call," I had just gotten through a *huge* hurdle of fear, and now, I could just lay there and count those wonderful, stained, square, dotted ceiling tiles.

Make That a Double

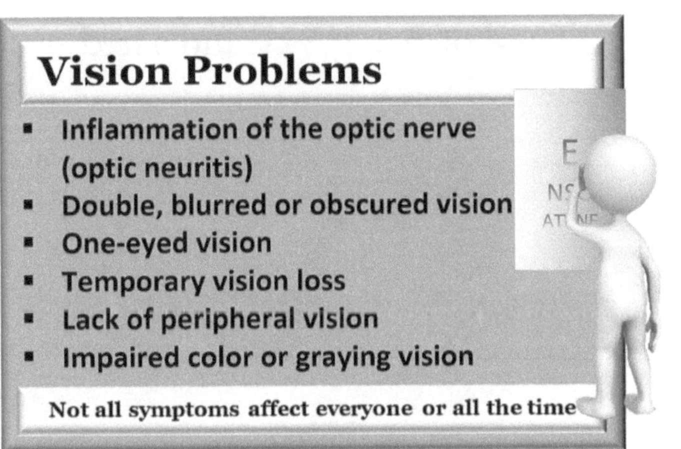

Recovery from the ruptured discs and subsequent surgery took months to return to previous activities. Though the injury had nothing to do with MS, the consequences of the ordeal had everything to do with it.

After surgery, I had increased seizures, exacerbated symptoms of all kinds, and soon afterward, a frightening stint of blurred, double vision so intense that for nearly two weeks I had to feel my way around the house. Like the beautiful partner that he is, Dennis drove me to and from work again never once complaining or giving the impression that he was "put out" in any way. Of course, he was worried, as was I, but dealing with random, unexplained issues for *years* had now become a routine part of both of our lives. With careful planning, I managed to hide the visual disturbance at work by focusing on writing/typing tasks that did not require clear vision. Thankfully, this diplopia ebbed away with not a soul at work aware of my struggle. In retrospect, I understand that I was experiencing an MS relapse, but at the time, I still didn't know I had MS.

Tired of Being Sick and Tired

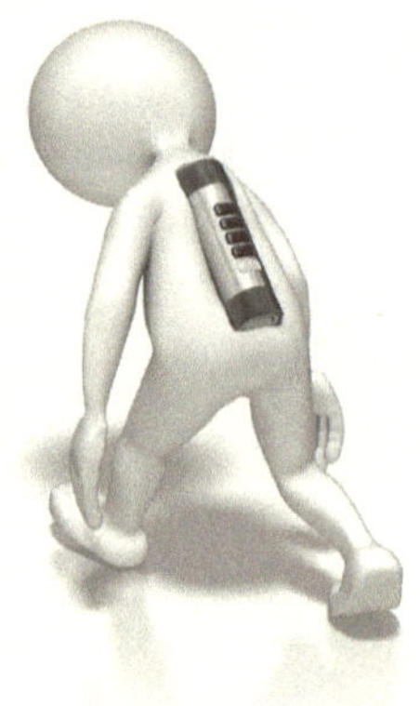

On anticonvulsants for over five years and still having random seizures and a myriad of other issues, I simply wasn't satisfied. How can an appropriate remedy be applied if I didn't know the cause? I was challenged with unexplained and intermittent symptoms and frustrated with how the anticonvulsants made me feel. Like a brainless mannequin in someone else's body, it was an ongoing struggle to feel or "act" normal when I felt so incredibly drained.

Maybe I would never find out, but suppose there was an underlying problem that *could* be identified? Suppose all the crazy symptoms were caused by these medications?

Suppose there was an explanation that didn't show early on but might be evident now? Was it reasonable to keep seeking answers, or was I to "give up," put my head in the sand and take these life-altering medications forever? *There had to be another way.*

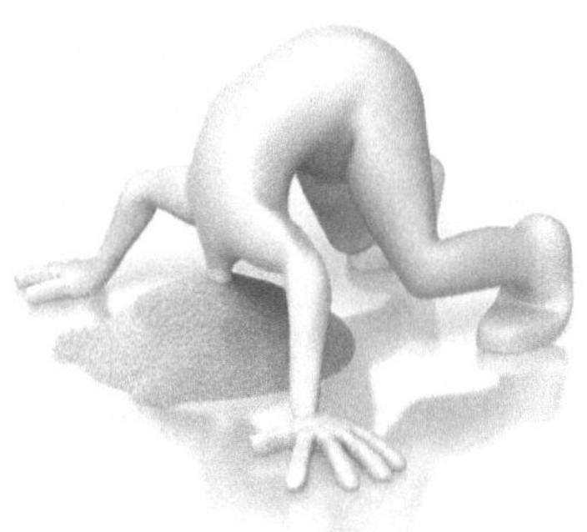

Frequently changing prescriptions due to toxicity or ineffectiveness, in five years, I had taken over a dozen different anticonvulsants. On several occasions, I needed emergency treatment to counteract adverse reactions to them. One day, while at work, my face swelled like a balloon. Fortunately, the surgeon I worked for took immediate action and had the nurse administer a shot and an antihistamine via IV to bring this allergic reaction under control. I saw my neurologist the next day.

Having switched from one "poison" to another during those five years, I'd had enough! It seemed my life consisted of going from work to bed to work to bed to work to bed … there was nothing left in me beyond that. I wanted my life back, and I'm sure my sweet, adoring, uncomplaining husband wanted his wife back! My wishes to get off these anticonvulsants were no secret to my neurologist. He did his best to find an anticonvulsant that my body would tolerate and would control the seizures. There was not a single visit that I didn't tell him how much I detested how these medications affected me.

I needed to know if the intermittent and random symptoms I was experiencing were related to the anticonvulsants, and I felt I would never know the answer to that question if I didn't find out for myself. During one particular visit, I told my neurologist that I'd had enough. I wanted off these medications. He warned me of possible consequences, the risks of worsening seizures and the dangers that could accompany that decision. His "pep talk" did not deter me. Knowing how adamant I was, he encouraged me to participate in the Epilepsy Program, a neurology center that specialized in seizure disorders. I was willing to try anything *except more medications!*

The Epilepsy Program

I was determined to do all I could to return to the life I knew before the flu, seizures, and other symptoms interrupted my "life as I knew it." The path I had been on those past five years was not accomplishing that goal. Although I knew nothing about this Epilepsy Program, I was willing to give it a try in hopes that the program might identify the root of the problem and hopefully offer a more effective solution.

My journey at the Epilepsy Program began with a simple, painless test called an EEG (electroencephalogram) that tracks and records the patterns of the brain's electrical impulses through small, flat metal electrodes that a technician adheres to the scalp. Each electrode has a wire attached at one end; the other end is connected to an instrument that amplifies and records the brain waves. The purpose of an EEG is to detect any abnormalities as well as the location of abnormal electric activity of the brain.

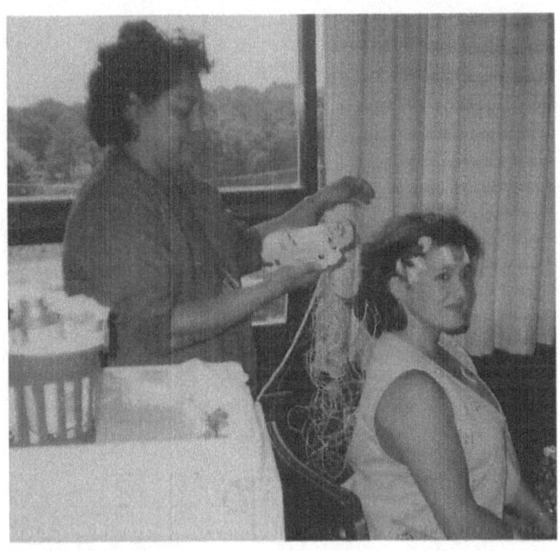

Allowed to sleep only between the hours of 2:00 to 5:00 a.m., sleep deprivation was used to bring on observable, recorded seizure activity. Thanks to the nightmarishly painful leg cramps (a result of abruptly taking me off anticonvulsants, which I'd been taking for five years), I was most assuredly sleep deprived. If I did start to doze, the neurology staff would communicate from the "command center" to the speakers in my room to ensure I remained awake (except during the allowed sleep hours.) If I showed signs of seizure activity, they checked on me or adjusted the electrodes.

The observation room was monitored twenty-four hours a day for the seven days I was there with the bathroom being the only location where I was not being "watched." I think it took a week *after* the program to get over the sense that I was still on camera being "watched."

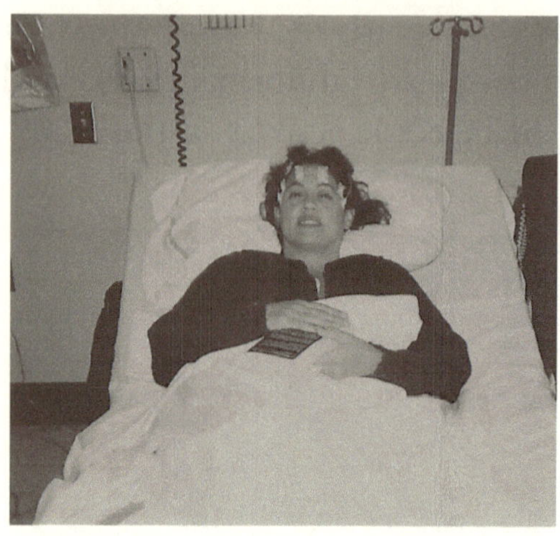

I had agreed to this madness not *really* knowing what I was getting into. I simply didn't want to take anticonvulsants any longer. By the end of this seven-day program, I was exhausted beyond description, and I swear I didn't gain a single thing by attending it. However, I was there for a reason, and my mission was accomplished. No more anticonvulsants!

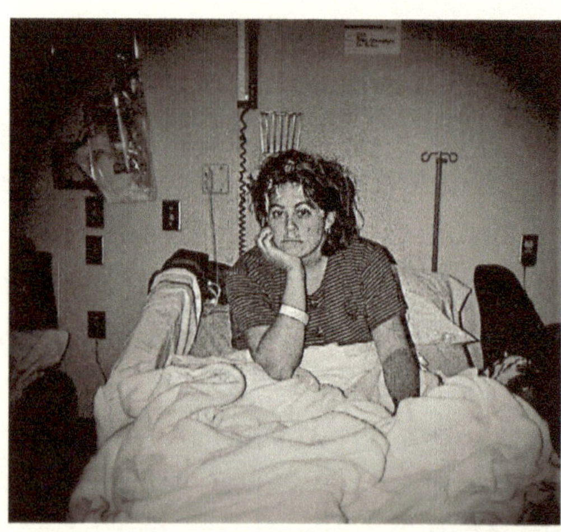

Initially, the neurologist at the Epilepsy Program did not support my request to discontinue anticonvulsants. I had already been through the ringer for a week getting off them, so I wasn't about to back down now. I explained emphatically that I was not planning to take these medications so would he please tell me what I needed to know. I think I may have even detected a shred of compassion somewhere behind that title as he saw I wasn't about to change my mind. He told me to monitor if I had worsening seizure activity, not to drive until I knew it was safe, and to stay in touch if needed.

As I look back on that decision, I see that, for me, it was a good one. No longer on anti-seizure medications, I had only occasional seizures (no more than when I was taking these meds.) I left the Epilepsy Program without a prescription, but I had gained a new problem—a sleep disorder that would follow me for well over a decade.

CHAPTER FOUR

Is Anybody Listening?

I had concluded that some unidentified neurological problem was the root of these ongoing issues since that flu in '97, but I would probably never know the cause. Nevertheless, over the years, I continued to mention specific struggles to my neurologist and physicians, and so it was that the symptoms described in this book were recorded in my medical records, yet nothing jumped out and screamed "multiple sclerosis." First of all, who reads *years* of past medical records? Doctors don't have time for that. I wasn't dying. I looked normal, I walked normal, I talked normal, and I acted normal (okay, I know, that's a subjective statement), but the bottom line is that while most of what I dealt with was "on again/off again," I was keenly aware that *something* was most assuredly "off."

Changing Direction

By 2010, new symptoms were greatly affecting me. I informed both my neurologist and my family doctor about increasing and painful leg spasms, inexplicable waves of intense fatigue, intermittent bouts of clumsiness and loss of balance, progressive hand weakness, and other sporadic and random issues. My greatest concern, however, had to do with memory issues, word retrieval challenges, and frequent struggles to get a thought from my mind out my mouth. I was really, *really* tired of bringing it up. I felt unheard and didn't know where to turn.

In 2011, symptoms were severe enough to re-evaluate the overall direction of my life and work. For those who have gone undiagnosed for long periods of time, you know what a struggle it is to *know* there's something amiss yet not know where else to turn for answers. After extended conversations with Dennis, we agreed it was time to make some changes. I submitted my resignation at work and left the outcome of our finances to the Lord. I never told a soul why I was resigning—I didn't know how. Although we still knew nothing about MS, we did know it was time to adjust my life to match the ongoing, progressing challenges.

A Different Approach

In 2012, in a desperate attempt to find answers, I explored options outside the usual medical community and scheduled an appointment with a naturopathic practitioner. Maybe a different perspective would offer some answers. I still had no idea I had MS—in fact, odd and random cognitive issues plagued me intermittently, and I started to wonder if I had Alzheimer's—that scary thought sparked my action for answers. I needed to get to the bottom of it.

As I had done many times before, I told this practitioner about the flu in '97 and the seizures and other symptoms that followed. She reviewed my medical history, and to rule out other infections or inflammation for which I had not been tested, she sent me for Western Blot Lyme and rheumatoid factor testing. When tests returned "within normal limits," she asked detailed questions and inquired if I'd had a brain MRI within the last five years. I had not. She also casually asked if the possibility of multiple sclerosis was ever brought up. Except for the Mayo Clinic years earlier when we were presented with the many possibilities that could affect a woman in her forties with symptoms and seizures like I had, MS was not mentioned. She recommended an MRI, and my family practitioner followed through with the referral without hesitation.

CHAPTER FIVE

"It" Has a Name

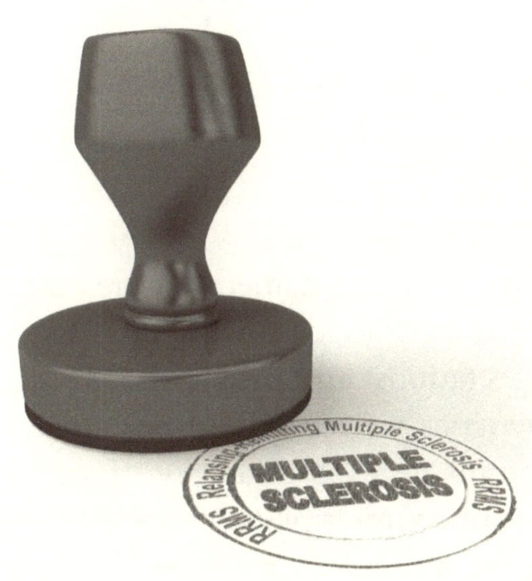

It was surreal to absorb the neurologist's words … "lesions … demyelination … *multiple sclerosis*." Well, well! "It" had a name. Yet surprisingly, *not knowing* what was going on all those years was far more exasperating than hearing the actual diagnosis. At least now, I had an answer.

That was a start. The words "relapsing-remitting multiple sclerosis" seemed a little ominous at first, but only because we didn't yet know much about it. Having a diagnosis brought a sense of relief; something *finally* made sense! I wanted to shout out loud to no one in particular (except maybe that endocrinologist from years gone by) "See! I'm *not* crazy!" (A tad ditzy? Yes. But crazy? No!)

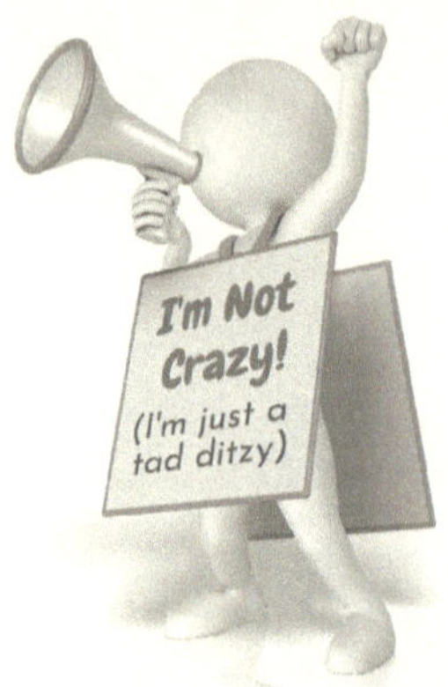

Now that "it" had a name, we were on a more defined quest to learn how to deal with this disease, treatment options, expectations, and prognosis. We shared scores of "aha" moments as we recognized how many long-experienced symptoms were "normal" and shared by many with relapsing-remitting multiple sclerosis (RRMS). The more we learned, the more empowered we became to deal with and accept it.

The following year, Dennis and I took steps to simplify our lives. It was an invigorating, exciting process. We moved closer to my son and his family and bought a new home with fewer demands, which allowed us more time with one another. We were taking control! Our decision proved to be a good one for us.

Just Curious

I have always wondered if and how that flu in '97 influenced or is related to having multiple sclerosis. In their book *Polymicrobial Diseases*, the authors explain that some MS patients may have had a *virus-induced disturbance that affected cells associated with the production of myelin in the central nervous system* that "might be the starting point for a subsequent switch to autoimmune demyelination." They write, "Recent pathological studies of MS strongly support the view of different pathogenic mechanisms as a first trigger of disease."[i]

The authors also write "in several studies, upper respiratory tract infections have been demonstrated to be related to an increased risk of both onset and exacerbations of MS."[ii]

Although I may never know with certainty the answer to why my brain went bonkers following that virus in 1997, articles such as these raise the possibility that, in my case, the onset of MS may have started with this flu. In my mind, there has *always* been a direct correlation to "life before and after" the flu and the seizures that followed.

In his article "Multiple Sclerosis: Can It Cause Seizures?" Dr. Mark Keegan (Mayo Clinic) states, "Epileptic Seizures are more common in people who have multiple sclerosis (MS) than those who don't ... Exactly why these seizures occur more in people with MS isn't completely understood. MS lesions in certain areas of the brain may trigger these seizures ... and may be the first noticeable sign of MS before diagnosis."[iii]

While there is no definitive trigger to MS, according to the National MS Society, exposure to certain microorganisms or common viruses during childhood raises the possibility that some "infectious agents or microorganisms such as measles, Epstein-Barr, Chlamydia pneumonia, human herpes virus-6 [HHV6], and other viruses may play a role in the development or in the triggering of MS.[iv]

The Multiple Sclerosis Association of America (MSAA) states, "Researchers have studied a variety of possible causes for multiple sclerosis (MS), and a combination of factors appears to be involved. A popular theory looks at commonly known *slow-acting viruses* (one that could remain dormant for many years), such as measles, herpes, human T-cell lymphoma, and Epstein-Barr. After being exposed to one of these viruses, some researchers theorize that MS may develop in *genetically susceptible people.*"[v]

Obviously, I'm not a microbiologist or medical professional, but I can't ignore data that may have contributed to setting me up as a candidate for multiple sclerosis. For example, my parents told me that when I was two years old, Mom went to get me from my crib and discovered my face contorted to one side so tightly I was unable to open one of my eyes. I was drooling profusely but smiling happily to get up from my nap. I was diagnosed with Bell's palsy. It took several months before the face drooping and drooling subsided.

What's that got to do with anything? Maybe nothing, but the Mayo Clinic writes: "Although the exact reason Bell's palsy occurs isn't clear, it's often linked to exposure to a viral infection" (such as) "herpes simplex, chickenpox and shingles (herpes zoster), mononucleosis (Epstein-Barr), Cytomegalovirus infections, respiratory illnesses (adenovirus), German measles (rubella), mumps virus, Flu (influenza B) … hand-foot-and-mouth disease (coxsackievirus)."[vi]

So there it is again—that Epstein-Barr virus popping its ugly little head out when I was only two.

At seventeen, I had mononucleosis, which kept me in bed for a solid *three months*. Not prone to doctor visits in those days, my mother brought me to our family physician *twice* as she was concerned about how long I was weak, fevered, and with swollen lymph nodes. I was so weak, in fact, Mom assigned my younger sister to care for me when I was alone.

The US National Library of Medicine National Institute of Health writes, "Infectious mononucleosis caused by the *Epstein-Barr virus has been associated with increased risk of multiple sclerosis*" (emphasis mine). The objective to one of their studies was to "assess the significance of sex, age at and time since infectious mononucleosis, and attained age to the risk of developing multiple sclerosis after infectious mononucleosis." They found "the risk of multiple sclerosis was persistently increased for more than 30 years after infectious mononucleosis."[vii]

It's all speculation, but I can't help but wonder if some common viruses (to which most people are exposed) didn't "set me up" for this disease. Not that it matters. Either way, I have it. I live with it. It's doable. Knowing or not knowing doesn't change a thing. I'm just curious.

CHAPTER SIX

MULTIPLE SCLEROSIS 101 (A SHORT EXPLANATION)

There is so much information "out there" that I do not want to appear to be an expert on the subject. I am not. But I do have relapsing-remitting multiple sclerosis, and I do understand how complex this disease can be, so I'll summarize the basics for those who may not understand it.

Multiple sclerosis is an "immune-mediated" disease in which one's own immune system attacks the *myelin*, the myelin-producing cells and/or underlying nerve fibers of the central nervous system (CNS).[viii]

Myelin works much like the rubber insulation covering conductor wires. "Electric hazards" or "misfires" exist when insulation is "frayed" or damaged. Helping to control and regulate the flow of electrical energy, myelin ensures that messages are contained and carried to the right places without interruption within the central nervous system. According to the National MS Society, because MS attacks cause scarring (sclerosis) of the myelin sheath (insulation), the nerve signals can encounter interruptions, distortions, or destruction to the impulses going to and from the spinal cord and brain.[ix]

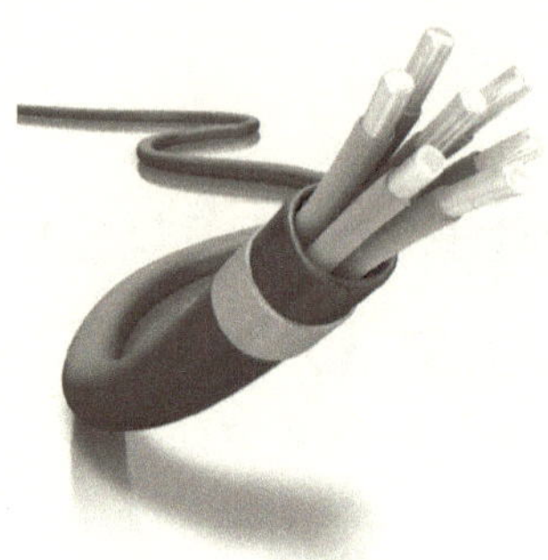

The central nervous system is responsible for guiding the movements of our bodies, for registering sensations that we feel, and for controlling our thought processes. Scarring of the myelin sheath can interfere with these nerve signals causing confusion to the impulses traveling to and from the CNS. Depending on how much or what area of the brain or spinal column is damaged, a long list of sporadic repercussions can ensue. These symptoms can appear isolated from each other, appear and disappear, and manifest singly or in combination over a period of many years and varies from person to person.

No wonder diagnosis of this disease is so perplexing!

Multiple sclerosis falls into three categories or "types." Knowing the type of MS you have can help you achieve a better understanding of how you may be affected.

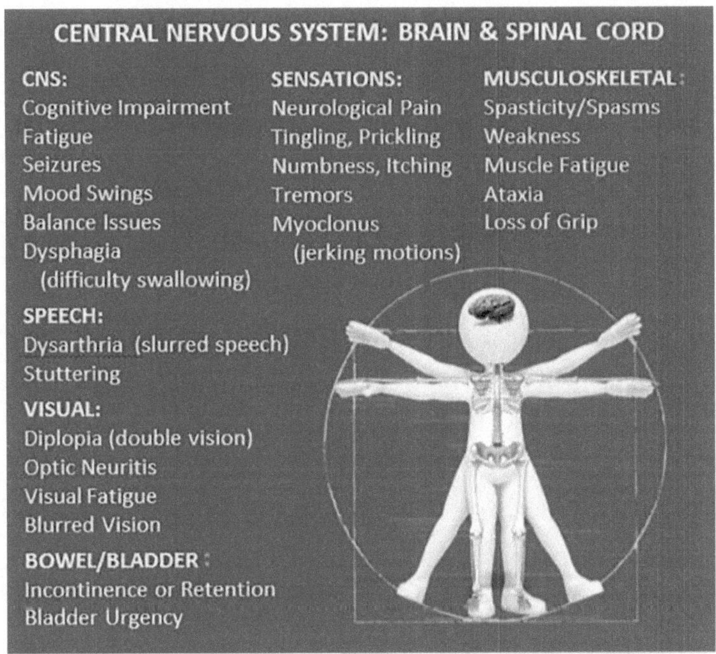

Relapsing/Remitting Multiple Sclerosis (RRMS)

According to the National MS Society, the most common type of MS, *relapsing-remitting multiple sclerosis* (RRMS), affects about 85 percent of everyone with this disease.[x]

Characterized by seemingly random attacks (relapses) where new or worsening conditions can last for weeks, months, or even longer, RRMS can range in severity, duration, and intensity from mild to severe. Relapses are commonly followed by periods of remission and stability where symptoms subside or even disappear. Some people have very few symptoms with long periods between setbacks. Others may experience frequent exacerbations of varying degrees. In either case, relapse can include a broad range of symptoms that vary greatly from person to person or relapse to relapse. With RRMS, some lingering symptoms may remain and relapses may become less frequent or even non-existent.

Secondary Progressive Multiple Sclerosis (SPMS)

In most cases of relapsing-remitting multiple sclerosis (about 90 percent), the disease itself can worsen to some degree over time with many symptoms eventually without remission. Some people may have more intense cognitive issues or mood swings, ongoing muscle spasticity or bladder issues, neurologically induced pain, or a host of other symptoms that progress unpredictably to some degree over time. Most RRMS cases become *secondary progressive multiple sclerosis (SPMS)*, which is often (though not always) more difficult to treat. It has also been observed that the older the patient when MS is diagnosed, the more likely he or she may be in the secondary progressive stage of MS due to years of myelin and nerve damage that occurred while yet undiagnosed.

According to Johns Hopkins Medicine, when the relapsing-remitting aspect of MS "changes to a point where there are no discernable relapses and remissions; the course of the disease has transitioned to *secondary progressive MS*." They explain how those with SPMS began with the RRMS course stating, "In secondary progressive MS, symptoms accumulate and worsen without any remission. There may be periods where symptoms are stable, but the overall course is one of worsening over time." Individuals describe changes "when comparing current function to past function but without identifying an episode that led to the worsening. Sometimes, after the onset of secondary progressive MS an individual may experience a relapse. The course would then be considered secondary progressive MS with relapses."[xi]

Like all stages of MS, *every person is different*. Individuals with SPMS may deal with specific symptoms that no longer go away and symptoms can vary in intensity from mild to severe depending on the extent and location of the nerve damage.

Primary Progressive Multiple Sclerosis

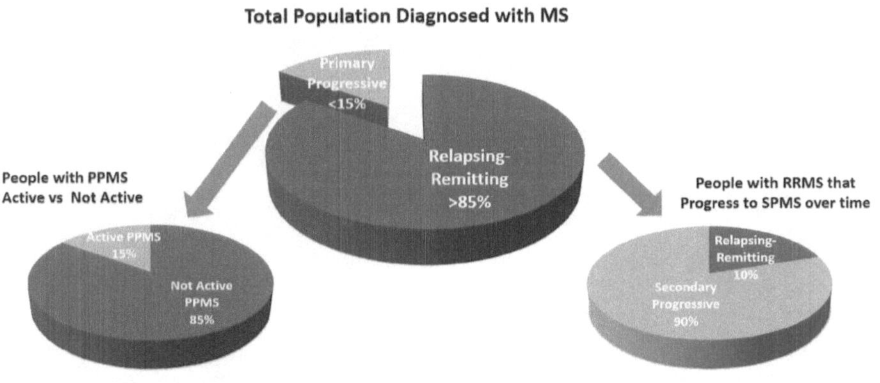

Fewer than 15 percent of people with MS are diagnosed with PPMS. Like other forms of MS, *primary progressive multiple sclerosis (PPMS)* affects each person to varying degrees and intensities. With PPMS, there is less actual inflammation and scarring of the *brain* than with the relapsing-remitting kind, but people with PPMS generally have increased lesions on the spinal cord and must face an unremitting decline of neurologic function. Nerve damage is the main issue with primary progressive MS, and it becomes progressively challenging for messages from the brain to make their way appropriately to other parts of the body such as the legs or hands. PPMS falls into one of two categories: it is either considered "active" or "not active."

Once the type of MS you have is identified, you can direct your research toward the most effective treatment for dealing with it.

CHAPTER SEVEN

MAKING SENSE OF SYMPTOMS

For those of us whose MS journey led us down countless and seemingly unrelated roads before diagnosis, we would attest that it was a multiyear, rabbit-chasing ordeal. Many of us had no idea that the years of diverse and sporadic symptoms were interconnected. Since diagnosis, however, I have found that I am one of *thousands upon thousands* with similar experiences.

Bizarre Symptoms

While each person with MS has a different list of symptoms that manifest either day to day, occasionally or ongoing, there is a commonality among us. *No two people with MS experience the same degree or intensity of symptoms or even the same symptoms.* Many may check the same boxes and/or add a few bizarre symptoms of their own. However, it's the same "monster." Symptoms vary according to the location of the lesions or amount of damage on the brain and/or central nervous system. Below are a few of the most common manifestations of multiple sclerosis—many I have never experienced, some I have experienced a few times or mildly, and others I experience more frequently. A few are an ongoing part of my life.

The Twilight Zone

Anyone can experience cognitive challenges from time to time and even more frequently as they age. However, "recall misfires" plague people with MS far more frequently than the general population in our age range. Less than 10 percent of the general population reports cognitive impairment. In comparison, as many as 65 percent of people with multiple sclerosis report mild to significant cognitive impairment. These challenges can be unpredictable and intermittent; they can pop in for a short time, linger, or seem they are here to stay, then vanish for a season; they can also be permanent. Such is the nature of the beast.

For many with MS, that all-too-frequent inability to recall what we were *just* talking about, the struggle with verbal fluency (the incapacity to find words at the tip of our tongues) or the inability to speak louder when we're told "you talk too softly" can be exasperating. We can fail to recall an event that *just* happened leaving us with a sense that we're living in the Twilight Zone. Don't ask me to tell you about a movie I saw last night or last week. That data is tucked away in a memory abyss and may or may not ever be retrieved. Recurrent "cognitive hiccups" are very much a part of MS.

It can sometimes seem that we are *almost* following along; in fact, if there was a "pause" button on actual conversations, we could "catch up." I've lost count how many times I have given Dennis "the look" because my brain is running two steps behind his words. We have developed an unspoken language between us with goofy faces and signals that mean "I'm not following you at all." No need to explain a thing—he just repeats what he said or slows down. Often, there's no recall, and all that's left is for us chuckle over it and move on … again.

If these misfires happen while with family or close friends or during an important conversation that we *really* need to follow (like getting directions, instructions, or signing a legal document), we may have to ask others to repeat what was said or invite the other party to slow down to allow our brain to process their words. The truth is that we *can* process *any* information, but not always in the timing of its output. It's one reason why texts, emails, and written reminders work so well for those who deal with these challenges. We can always go back and read the message again (and again) until it sinks in.

Bear in mind that many other factors such as stress or certain medications can cause cognitive issues for *anybody*; however, for those with MS, lesions are likely the culprit. We'd *love* to get a "faster hard drive" in this brain of ours, but until there is a cure for MS, we're pretty much stuck with what we have and must learn to find ways to adjust to this deficit. Ideas for addressing cognitive issues are covered in the chapter "Confronting the Giant."

See You Next Fall …

Many times, in the course of the day, I experience a sense that I'm falling. To manage this experience, I generally "hang out" by a wall, chair, countertop, or any reference point with which to make contact and keep me "grounded." It can be a challenge to experience a multitude of random sensations. We can't always discern if they are actual or "phantom" sensations. The sense that we are falling (whether we are really falling, or our sensory perception just makes it feel like we're falling) has the same impact on us as we react to "catch" ourselves.

There is a long list of sensations that can plague individuals with MS, many are covered in more detail in this book including burning sensations, pins and needles, itching or tingling, crawling sensations, hypersensitivity to touch (so sensitive that even the bed sheets or our clothing can "hurt"), a sense that the ground or the bed under us is "rumbling" on one or both sides of our body, and that unsettling sense that we are falling forward or backward.

Dizziness or Vertigo

- False sense that the world is spinning
- Very common symptom of MS
- Frequent sense of loss of balance
- Lightheadedness
- Feels like you're about to fall
- Can affect gait or the ability to walk without assistance

Not all symptoms affect everyone or all the time

I often remind friends and family that if they're going to hug me, they need to not just "let go" following that hug, or I could fall forward or backward. I remind them during a hug, "Okay, so let me catch my balance before you let go!" Because the messages from the brain to the central nervous system experience disruptions, there are many challenges such as this that others may not realize. *It's up to us to tell them.*

Too Hot to Trot

I have *really* struggled with heat sensitivity for many years. It was easy to blame it on menopause and hormones, and undoubtedly, they played a role at one point. However, I have learned to recognize that for me, heat is a powerful provoker of MS symptoms.

Heat or Cold Sensitivity

- Heat/Cold sensitivity very common in MS
- Frequent feelings of being extremely hot or cold (symptoms exacerbated by heat or cold)
- Extreme fluctuations in body temperature can worsen cognition, concentration and memory

Not all symptoms affect everyone or all the time

Surprisingly, up to 80 percent of people with MS deal with excessive heat (or cold) sensitivity—a condition that causes exacerbation of other symptoms such as fatigue, pain, or cognitive malfunctions. When our core body temperature increases *even slightly* (due to warmer weather, physical exercise, illness, stress, or being in an environment that challenges our personal MS—internal thermostat), it often results in worsening MS symptoms until that core temperature returns to what is tolerable to each individual. Heat or cold can disrupt messages to and from the brain and central nervous system and wreak all kinds of havoc. Some individuals with MS may experience visual symptoms (Uhthoff's phenomenon) or various other symptoms when they are overheated. Many have found that the use of cooling products such as misting fans, cooling vests, cooling neck wraps, ice packs and cold drinks are "must have handy" items to help us endure over-exposure to heat and enable us to enjoy more outdoor activities on hot days.

While increased core temperature does not cause additional nerve damage, it can and does make MS symptoms more intense for many individuals. Cold weather can also affect people with MS, causing exacerbated spasticity, stiffness, pain, and other symptoms. Many are affected by both excessive heat *and* cold.

Exaggerated heat/cold sensitivity can be a challenge when others may not understand how temperature can have consequences on people with MS. I used to avoid situations that would inconvenience others or put me at risk of overheating. However, I've found a happy medium. In my own home, I maintain the temperature I need, but I also keep jackets and blankets handy for cold-natured guests. In environments I can't control, when available, I drink ice water and use the glass to cool my face, or I go outside to cool down if needed. A personal misting fan can be a godsend, and if all else fails, if I must leave because my internal temperature is out of control, I do. What I don't do anymore, however, is isolate myself because of MS symptoms.

Wrong Pipe

When swallowing issues are problematic, it can make us a little timid about eating in public or around people we don't know well.

There have been many times that the food I was attempting to swallow came out my nostrils in a most embarrassing display. You know what it's like when food or drink "goes down the wrong pipe"? It feels like that, only choking can occur with or without food or drink. When I started choking for no apparent reason, I was forced to seek medical advice. First, I asked my pharmacist if any of my prescriptions might have this side effect; he reviewed and said no.

Swallowing Difficulties

- Dysphagia (difficulty swallowing)
- Can occur in any stage of MS but more often with advanced MS
- Frequent choking on food or drink
- Choking when laughing, talking, or for no apparent reason
- Silent aspiration

Not all symptoms affect everyone or all the time

Then I asked my doctor, "Doc, could I choke to death when this happens? Or would I just pass out and my throat would open? I don't want a prescription or anything, I just want to know what I'm dealing with here!"

I had already had an endoscopy earlier in the year which showed no issues. Yet I could be sipping a cup of coffee, chatting with friends, eating dinner, singing, reading, folding laundry, or just "sitting there" when suddenly, without provocation, I would just choke—I mean really *choke*. It felt like I "half swallowed" and my throat was closed. I was without air and couldn't breathe in or out until the muscle in my throat "released," then a tiny air hole opened, and I'd be gasping air with all my might. My doctor explained "dysphagia" and how it can occur at any or several different phases of the swallowing process (oral, pharyngeal, or esophageal phases.) He also explained that with MS, dysphagia can come and go and that it's not unusual to have swallowing issues for days, weeks, or even months, and just as quickly as it starts, the issue can disappear. Fortunately for me, at least as of this writing, the frequency of choking is more "occasional." Welcome to the sporadic, unpredictable world of relapsing/remitting multiple sclerosis!

For those who have a continued problem with swallowing or choking, a "swallow study" can help identify at which phase of the swallowing process the problem occurs. If you experience swallowing difficulties, other factors nonrelated to MS can also be the cause. Talk to your doctor to ensure there are no other issues masquerading as MS. My doctor referred me to a cognitive/speech therapist who showed me exercises and techniques to deal with swallowing issues when they manifest—I still do these exercises even if the problem is dormant.

The "Puppet Pull"

There is a sensation I use to call "*The Puppet Pull*" long before I was diagnosed with MS. I remember being *so* miserable at work with this squeezing sensation I knew nothing about. There was no position or posture that could ease the inexplicable tightness around my ribs and torso. I described it to Dennis as feeling "like a puppet being squeezed from the inside out." It is sometimes felt in the middle or sides of my back, but it can be felt in the chest too. Many describe it like an "elastic band pulling tightly around the torso." It is a truly miserable, distracting, and debilitating sensation and can feel like breathing is a task. When that tightness is present, I don't really want to tote a boa constrictor with me to do anything or go anywhere. The sensation is exhausting, so I give myself permission to "veg-out" and do nothing until it passes. It can last hours, days, or intermittently for weeks.

As with other symptoms, not everyone with MS experiences this sensation. For me, when it is present, it can be one of the worse symptoms of MS. This "hug" occurs when the intercostal muscles between the ribs tighten (like a spasm). Who knew I would later learn that even *that* miserable sensation had a name: the *"MS Hug"*. This is one hug I would gladly do without!

What a Jerk

Myoclonus (involuntary jerking or twitching of a muscle or muscle group) affects everyone from time to time. Hiccups are a type of myoclonus as are hypnic jerks that sometimes happen when drifting off to sleep. While scientists don't fully understand myoclonus, they believe it occurs when the part of the brain that controls movement is overexcited. When there is an underlying neurological disorder in the nerves or brain (such as with Parkinson's, Alzheimer's, epilepsy, multiple sclerosis, etc.) myoclonus can occur randomly, when at rest, any time of day or night, one time, frequently and with or without a pattern.

Tremors, Jerking

- Involuntary muscle twitching, shaking, jerking, tics or tremors
- Myoclonus "startled-like" motions
- Resting tremors (greatest when at rest)
- Postural tremors (greatest when sitting or standing)
- Intention tremors (greatest when moving)

Not all symptoms affect everyone or all the time

Others (hopefully) don't notice that sometimes we may sit on our hands because this crazy "jerking" motion is not only distracting to ourselves, but it can make us quite self-conscious if we're in an environment where it's difficult to hide. I have literally hit myself in the face while falling asleep or minding my own business quietly reading a book. Without warning, an arm or leg will straighten out and become rigid as a tree trunk. For me, myoclonus is more common when my body is at rest. My hands, legs, arms, head, feet, eyes, lips, face, or limbs can "twitch" randomly, or one or more body parts may downright jerk. I have learned to live with it or not even notice or care when it happens when I'm home with Dennis, but if I'm with others who may not understand MS, it's far more distracting and uncomfortable.

While these jerking/twitching movements are pain-less, they are also unpredictable in intensity or frequency although sometimes it seems more prevalent than others. Myoclonus can manifest as what some MS'ers call "jumps." It can be so intense that the jerking movement can literally cause the body (or an arm or leg) to suddenly become rigid so swiftly that some people have said they were "jerked" right out of their seats. Seriously! What a jerk!

Too Pooped to Pop

Fatigue

- Affects >80% of people with MS
- Often Interferes with ability to function
- Tends to worsen as day progresses
- Total exhaustion can occur suddenly and without warning
- Aggravated by heat or humidity
- Many with MS affected daily by fatigue

Not all symptoms affect everyone or all the time

Affecting at least 80 percent of people with MS, fatigue can be a real game changer. We never know how full our "energy bank" will be on any given day or when it will run out. I can go weeks or even months with a normal amount of energy. However, for most of us, there is usually no warning—we go from having energy to having *none!* Fatigue can strike like a meteorite leaving us barely able to walk back to the car without using the shopping cart as a "walker." Everything from balance to vision to strength to memory can be adversely affected, and all we can think about is *how fast can we get home!*

For example, on any given day, I can wake up refreshed and energetic. I'm a habitual "list maker" and can have a long growing list of errands I set out to complete. I'm feeling great; I feel *normal!* I map my day's journey so I can be frugal with my energy rations and regularly avoid large department stores that consume too much of my "energy reserves." Not an hour into errands—BAM—*just like that,* my energy bank can be depleted leaving me physically bankrupt with my body in foreclosure. When this happens, it takes everything in me to stand in line to cash out, pile my purchases into the car and drive home. Functioning on "overload" to carry the sacks inside, I put away food that could perish without refrigeration and leave the rest on the counter until later. *This* kind of fatigue can drop us like a sack of potatoes!

Bite Me

Remember as a kid when you'd sit on your foot in class, daydreaming, forgetting you were in school because there was a pigeon perched on the window sill calling your attention, or the wind was bending the trees outside, or a butterfly flew by and took your imagination on its wings? (Oh, come on, don't tell me you never did that!) Suddenly the foot you were sitting on became crazy numb with a weird "tingly" sensation that felt like little ants biting. (You *do* know what I'm talking about, right?)

Even as I type, today, I have that numb/tingling sensation in my left hand that has nagged and distracted me on and off for several days. It comes uninvited and unprovoked and goes away just as suddenly. Sometimes, it feels like just one hand is *freezing*; like I've been making snowballs without mittens—yet it's warm to the touch. *That's* what this numbness and tingling feels like.

Unless you are "blessed" with this curse, you can't know how much thought and effort is sometimes exerted trying to sit still or maintain attention. That annoying, prickly, itching sensation in our legs or feet or arms or hands (or nose or face or inner ear, or …) makes sitting through a meeting, a sermon at church, or a laid-back movie with friends a mild form of torture. It can sometimes be just plain distractingly miserable and can disappear just as suddenly as it appeared—without warning or without reason.

Down and Out

I'm a "glass half full" kind of person and have never had to deal with clinical depression. I did, however, have a taste of depression when a medication prescribed for sleep brought an ominous "dark cloud" over me. As soon as I recognized it, I stopped taking it, and that sense of gloom and doom disappeared. I am thankful for that short but intense bout of depression. It gave me compassion for those who deal with depression as part of their everyday lives.

Depression

- **Can be MS-related neuroendocrine or immune system changes that affect mood**
- **Can be side effect of MS-related meds**
- **Can be from emotional challenge in dealing with loss of function or abilities**
- **Seek help with depression if needed**

Not all symptoms affect everyone or all the time

While stress, medications, and external factors may contribute to feelings of depression, multiple sclerosis itself can also be the cause. When there is scarring (sclerosis) to the myelin sheath that insulates and protects your nerves, mood signals can be distorted and send messages that your brain interprets as depression. You are not imagining these feelings, and *it's not your fault*. Don't feel embarrassed, weak, or ashamed that MS may have emotional, physiological, and psychological effects on you.

If depression is a problem, don't deal with it alone. Talk to your doctor. Talk to someone who understands MS, and if you don't feel there is anyone listening, contact the National MS Society—they have an online chat that can answer questions: http://www.nationalmssociety.org/Resources-Support, and if needed contact the suicide prevention life line at 800.273.8255 or visit their website for the chat link: https://suicidepreventionlifeline.org/

Lost in Space

While there are some people (like Dennis) who have an innate sense of direction no matter where they are, there are others (like myself) who live with their car in "reverse" due to a *very* poor sense of direction. A "bad sense of direction" is, for many, quite normal. The article *Why Do You Always Get Lost* explains that a complex structure within the brain called the hippocampus holds unique neurons that generate a "cellular map" that helps us classify spatial awareness—these neurons (called grid cells) also play a huge role in helping us recognize not only where we've been and where we are, but also where we're going.[xii] It's a highly useful tool that seems to work in varying degrees for different people with or without MS.

So while I am one who has *never* had a good sense of direction, I also have a ridiculous, intermittent, and seemingly nonexistent sense of direction that has plagued me and frequently left me with the inability to sense where I am. I am completely dependent on "exit" signs to find my way out of buildings, and GPS is one of my best friends. In the article "Common Multiple Sclerosis-Related Cognitive Problems," the author shares how MS affects visual perceptual skills such as simple perception, recognition of objects, or our sense of direction and orientation in space and how these challenges can interfere with activities such as reading a map, driving, programming the VCR, or dealing with "those pesky 'some assembly required' projects."[xiii]

Most people know what it's like to be "turned around," but many with MS experience what it's like to be turned around and around and then flipped upside down! It's a challenge to live in a world that seems to be constantly changing direction on us, and we must do our best to get around in it. Personally, I can't fully blame MS for my poor sense of direction, but it is a prime suspect regarding how much worse it is now than it used to be. The old saying, "she can't find her way out of paper bag" is, for me, all too true.

Spatial Disorientation

Spatial Orientation Challenges

- Compromised spatial awareness (dysmetria)
- Difficulty judging distance of a specific target
- Under-reaching or over-reaching for an object
- Loss of coordination in movement

Not all symptoms affect everyone or all the time

Remember all those goofy-seeming tests at the neurology clinic where you were asked to touch your nose then the doctor's moving finger? Or you were instructed to stand with your feet together, arms extended, palms up with your eyes closed (is that even possible?), then, without warning, the doctor gave you an unexpected "shove"? Or while sitting there, with his hand on the back of your head, the neurologist quickly pushed your head forward toward your chest. How about the scrape-the-pen-tip-up-the-sole-of-your-foot test? That one can be a toe curling doozie! Many other seemingly random actions and tests performed during a neurological assessment have made us ask ourselves, "What was *that* about?"

Each of these actions performed during a neurological exam has a specific purpose that tests the cranial nerves and visual fields, the motor system and reflexes, the sensory system and coordination, position sense, gait testing, and more. For example, the finger-to-nose test can help the neurologist determine if a patient may have compromised spatial awareness (AKA dysmetria) that can result in poor hand-eye coordination, misjudging how far away an object is, difficulty in picking up objects, or under- or overshooting the reach of a hand, arm, leg or eye. In MS, dysmetria is usually caused by lesions in the area of the brain responsible for coordinating movement (the cerebellum) and affects one's ability to accurately judge distance or scale. Not all in-office neurological tests contribute to the diagnosis of MS, but they are several of the many basic tests that can reveal abnormalities that help with diagnosis.

Balance Issues

Balance can be adversely affected when messages to and from the brain and central nervous system (CNS) are not transported fast enough or to the right place. Balance problems can stem from dizziness or vertigo as well as from other factors—but no matter the cause, it certainly affects walking, standing still, or the ability to remain upright when moving or when navigating from one type of surface to another (i.e., carpet to tile, concrete to grass, flat ground to incline.)

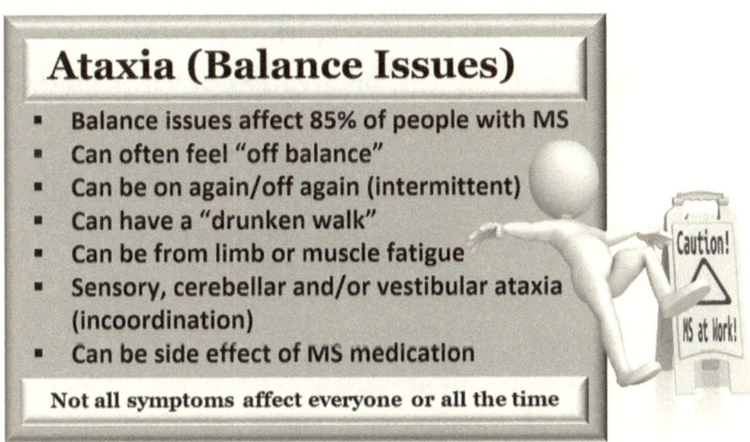

In one study, *MS in America*, the survey showed that, "91% (n=3,009) of participants said that they experienced difficulties with walking, balance, or coordination and 49% (n=3,132) noted these problems as their most significant initial MS symptoms. Muscle weakness and loss of balance were the two most common symptoms associated with walking, balance, & coordination problems."[xiv]

For many, balance issues can come and go without warning, vary day to day, or stay long term. It can affect people with MS differently and vary in intensity and duration or become a permanent part of someone's life. There are many contributing factors to balance problems, which can be directly related to MS lesions, a side effect of medications, inner ear issues, visual disturbances, numbness, and other factors relating to the brain and central nervous system.

When MS lesions affect our equilibrium (that state of stability where opposing forces like gravity and your own ability to provide postural control and spatial orientation through your senses) and/or proprioception (our awareness of where our body is in relation to the environment we are in), our sense of balance can be greatly compromised.

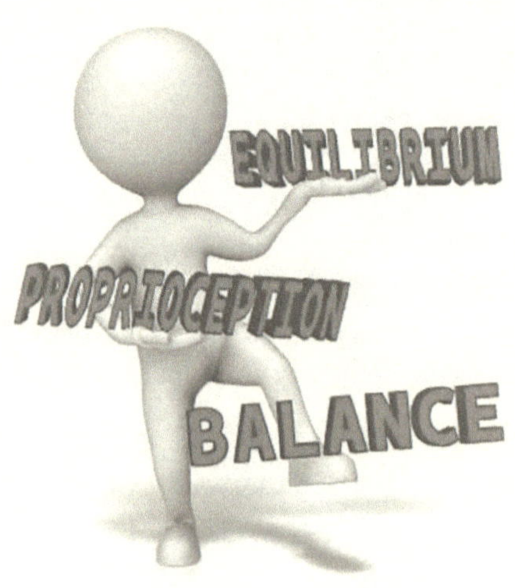

When our ability to readily process messages from the brain and central nervous system is interrupted, slowed down, or conflicting, it's easy to see why MS can sometimes feel like a roller coaster ride with unexpected dips, falls, twirls, and may even, at times, leave us feeling a bit nauseous!

Don't Say the "S" Word!

No one likes to talk about this one, but let's be honest here—when the central nervous system is affected, then so is sexual response. Fatigue and pain can hinder intimacy, and random interrupted nerve impulses can also affect sexual responsiveness. Those moments when there *is* a spark that turns to a flame, nothing extinguishes a romantic moment faster than a full fledge, impossible-to-ignore, downright painful whole leg and buttock muscle spasm.

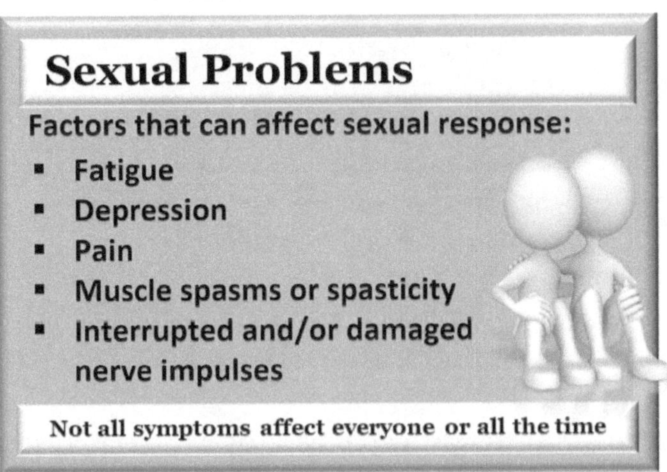

When the "reward" for sexual intimacy is a simultaneous charley horse so intense that it "changes the subject" faster than you can say, "Oh, baby," your intimate life is definitely affected. This kind of pain can instill a little "fear" and apprehension in what should be a glorious moment. Of course, MS is not the only cause of these symptoms, but it is certainly a common one.

That Smarts!

Some people with MS claim they experience no pain at all. However, chronic pain affects 55 percent to 65 percent of people with MS to varying degrees and is often a regular part of our everyday lives. If we complained every time we had a random, shooting, stabbing electrical-shock-like current of pain we would be squealing often and throughout the day like baby piglets looking for their momma.

Random/ Chronic Pain

- MS-related pain affects 55-65%
- Can be random, shooting pain
- Can be acute or chronic
- Can be felt anywhere in the body
- Spasms/Spasticity in any muscle group
- Musculoskeletal, paroxysmal or chronic neuropathic pain

Not all symptoms affect everyone or all the time

There are different categories of MS-related pain that can be sporadic and intermittent or acute and chronic and can be felt anywhere in the body.

Musculoskeletal pain (also known as "secondary pain") is not caused directly by MS itself but usually brought on by MS symptoms. For example, inactivity, spasticity, and compromised posture can cause musculoskeletal pain; balance issues can produce secondary pain in the hip, ankle, and knee joints due to joint compromise trying to maintain balance.

Because maintaining balance is a challenge, our bodies overcompensate to keep us upright. The overcompensation places unnatural strain on our joints. If we've been on our feet for long periods of time without something to keep us stable (a cane, walker, grocery cart, someone's arm), we may pay for it with hours-long muscle spasms or spasticity, or other hip, foot or ankle maladies. If progressive MS has forced an individual in fixed positions, he or she may have secondary pain due to inactivity in the muscles or ligaments.

Unlike musculoskeletal pain, *neuropathic pain* is more directly related to MS itself. When the central nervous system malfunctions, it can cause honest-to-goodness, not-in-your-head acute or chronic neuropathic *pain*, which can affect multiple areas of the body simultaneously. This type of pain is difficult to describe but is often compared to a "toothache-like" pain anywhere in the body. Others describe it as burning, intense aching, or a sensation of uncomfortable pressure—all of which can vary in intensity and get worse or better for no known reason and be unpredictable in duration.

Neuropathic pain occurs when damaged nerves become hypersensitive sending pain signals when there isn't an actual injury. Some describe it as "an illusion" created by the misfiring of signals within the central nervous system. It is a very *real* pain and for many, it is something we live with every day of our lives.

Merriam-Webster defines paroxysmal as "a fit, attack, or sudden increase in recurrence of symptoms … a sudden violent emotion or action." With MS, there are many symptoms that come on suddenly as "attacks"—they may last seconds, minutes, hours, or even days, but they come on with a vengeance and disappear just as suddenly. This type of pain can come in cycles, happen only once, repeat just a few times, or occur multiple times in one day. Some call them "surges" or "episodes," but this random "out of nowhere" paroxysmal pain is common with MS and includes spasms, some vision issues, "ice pick" pain or what I call "lightning jolts."

Paroxysmal Symptoms

- Symptoms that recur or intensify suddenly and without warning (spasms, seizures)
- Can manifest as "hot flashes", flutter of lip or eyelid, or sudden intense shooting pain in eye, face, or extremities
- Can be triggered by fatigue, sudden shift in body posture, elevation of core temperature
- Sometimes a sign of impending relapse

Not all symptoms affect everyone or all the time

When we "EEK" out of nowhere because a "lightning jolt" just surged through our face or feet or eye or hand, or a muscle spasm grips us in the middle of our sleep and doesn't let up, believe us, we aren't "making something out of nothing."

Hold That "Thought!"

Once upon a time, I didn't know the meaning of the words "bladder urgency" or "overactive bladder"; those were the "good ol' days" before aging *and* MS got hold of my bladder and shook the living daylights out of it.

Anyone with bladder urgency or overactive bladder understands the "pee-pee dance." One second we're standing near the sink rinsing dishes—the next we are *running* to the toilet as fast as we can. By now, we have learned *not* to close the toilet seat because that one extra second can mean … well … too late! We learn to empty the bladder before running errands, not drink while out and take full advantage of the restrooms before embarking on errands away from home. Welcome to the world of multiple sclerosis and compound that even greater if you're over sixty!

Bladder Control Issues

- Often MS-related due to nerve damage
- Bladder urgency
- Overactive bladder
- Loss of bladder control
- Inability to fully empty bladder
- Prone to urinary tract infections (UTIs)
- Bladder incontinence

Not all symptoms affect everyone or all the time

For many with MS, an inability to empty the bladder completely is a challenge. UTIs (urinary tract infections) are not uncommon with MS, and to the dismay of many, neither is bladder incontinence. Don't just "give up" on that overactive bladder though—physical therapy can help tremendously. Others have found natural remedies helpful in reducing bladder urgency or incontinence, and if natural remedies don't work, there are prescription medications for this problem as well.

Although most people with MS do not have bowel problems, there are some with MS that must deal with it. Bowel problems include constipation (often induced by certain medications or inactivity), a slowed digestive tract, decreased movement through the intestines, or loss of bowel control. The good news is that in most cases, bowel issues can be controlled through diet, supplements and, if needed, prescription medications.

Which remedy should you consider for your bladder or bowel issues? I guess I'd have to say, it "Depends."

Catch Me Some Zs Please!

I have a personal routine to "celebrate" sleep that includes a relaxing bath, my essential oil diffuser with lavender and other oils that promote relaxation, the thermostat set cool enough to match my heat-intolerance levels (which are more sensitive at night), running the ceiling fan, incorporating "white noise" in the room, turning off any lights, and playing my online Bible or some quiet music. Yes, I really do this *every* night because sleep is something I have to *work* for. After years of sleep deprivation following that stay in the Epilepsy Program, I take sleep very seriously and have managed to catch some "Zs" without the use of any prescription drugs. My recommendation is to find what works and do it! Sleep is important to our health and well-being.

There is much discussion regarding the use of the cannabis herb and its potential benefits or risks for certain neurological disorders. The National Multiple Sclerosis Society provides excellent information on this topic including information from the American Academy of Neurology (a group of neurologist and neuroscientists who evaluate complementary and alternative medicine [CAM] for people with nervous system disorders.)[xv] The Multiple Sclerosis Society also has an excellent article "Five Myths About Cannabis and MS," which provides useful information on this topic.[xvi] Most importantly, as with any decision you make regarding your health, *do your homework!*

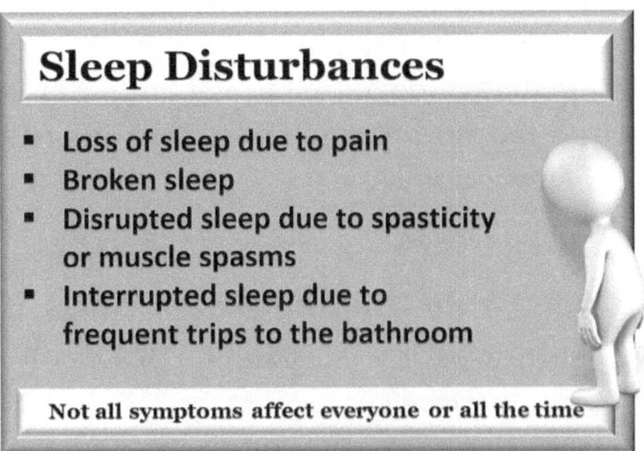

"BOO!"

I have nearly hit the ceiling when all Dennis did was clear his throat. An exaggerated startle response is not uncommon in people with MS. Triggered by sudden moves, unexpected actions, or loud noise, the "surprise response" can sometimes be a bit of a nuisance.

One time, when at the movie theater with my family, my grandson whispered, "Mema, you're not going to scream during this movie, are you?" Trust me, he had good reason to ask this question! I have been known to ignite a domino effect of "screamers" that reacted to *my* reaction during a surprise scene in a movie. So in answer to his question, umm … yeah, if the noise is sudden and loud or there is an unexpected scene that sparks my "surprise" response I *will* react, and likely it will be with a body jolting, short-lived, ridiculously loud scream. But it's not on purpose, and it can't be stopped. It's an involuntary, exaggerated startle response, which is common in people with MS, and it doesn't just happen "at the movies." If you don't like attention drawn to yourself in the middle of an intense moment in a theater full of people, don't invite me to go with you. *I even scare myself!*

Exaggerated Startle Response

- Sudden muscle contractions (myoclonus)
- Can develop in people with MS
- Stimulus-sensitive myoclonus can be triggered by sudden moves or loud noise
- Resembles "surprise response"

Not all symptoms affect everyone or all the time

If I Had a Hammer …

Headaches or migraines are twice more common in people with MS than in the general public. While not a common symptom, migraines are often among the first reported symptoms of MS. It doesn't matter if a symptom is "common" or not when it's affecting *you*.

The possibility that certain foods, medications, or other factors not related directly to MS could be responsible for these symptoms is certainly worth exploring and discussing with your medical team.

CHAPTER EIGHT

MANAGING INVISIBLE SYMPTOMS

Invisible symptoms present their own unique problems to our psyche as well as to our bodies. Because many symptoms are invisible to others, we may disqualify ourselves from admitting that we're struggling or seeking treatment that may help manage symptoms.

I'm sure you have already found that people are often surprised to learn you have MS. It's common to hear *"You have MS? Well, we could never tell! You look like you're doing great!"* They may then go on to tell us all about their cousin or neighbor or someone they know that's been in a wheelchair for thirty years. That's okay! I'm thankful MS does not affect me to that extent, and I hope it never does. I also know that they have *no* idea how MS does affect us in so many ways. They can't know. They don't live in our bodies, so when someone shares their opinion, I just nod my head and smile.

Momentum Magazine, the magazine of the National MS Society, has an excellent article entitled *Invisible Symptoms in MS: how to help others "see" Your Symptoms—and How They*

Affect You.[xvii] The article points out that "It's also important to use examples when discussing your symptoms … when people with MS tell someone they're fatigued, they often get responses like, 'Oh, I get tired, too' … to help someone understand MS fatigue, use phrases like 'my legs feel heavy' or 'lifting my hair dryer feels like I'm lifting a 25-pound weight.'"

The author shares another example when explaining how issues affect us. "To help her husband understand how her cognition and fatigue issues are affecting her at a specific time, she told her husband 'When I was driving today, I got so tired I couldn't find my way home. And I couldn't focus enough to understand what the woman was saying on the GPS.'" *How well I can understand this statement!*

For those of us who deal with MS, we are keenly aware that our symptoms are *very* real and can affect our everyday lives, our social interactions, and at times, dictate how or if we can accomplish anything today. On a good day, most anything can be a breeze; on a bad day, putting one lead-heavy foot in front of the other is almost more than we can muster. Some may now contend with long-term issues that no longer remit and must deal with compromised ability to do things we once loved.

At one time, the dust on my guitar reminded me that some things are now just a very happy memory of days gone by. It wasn't all that long ago that putting my guitar away in its case felt like I'd given up (although I knew someday I'd just be tired of dusting it.) When I faced reality, I handed my well-used, vintage, twelve-string Ovation guitar to my eldest son, Brandon (a music and worship leader at his church); I passed my father's beloved, antique banjo to my son Derek, and I gave my music binder to my daughter, April. It made my heart glad to take them off the shelves, out of the closet and into the care of my children who would appreciate and use them more than I could, and it felt good to purge my house of "stuff" I could no longer use. I have picked up new hobbies over the years that better match my abilities, and I am happy with these changes. Why focus on any disabilities when so many more good things await to be discovered and unleashed?

CHAPTER NINE

TELLING OTHERS

Telling others that you have MS can be awkward and difficult especially if many of your symptoms are invisible to others. It certainly takes courage to do so, but bear in mind that there are elements of telling others that you will want to consider—such as *who* to tell, *what* to tell them, *why* tell anyone at all, and *how* to tell others. I had to face these questions and answer them for myself to move on to the next stage of … well … moving on!

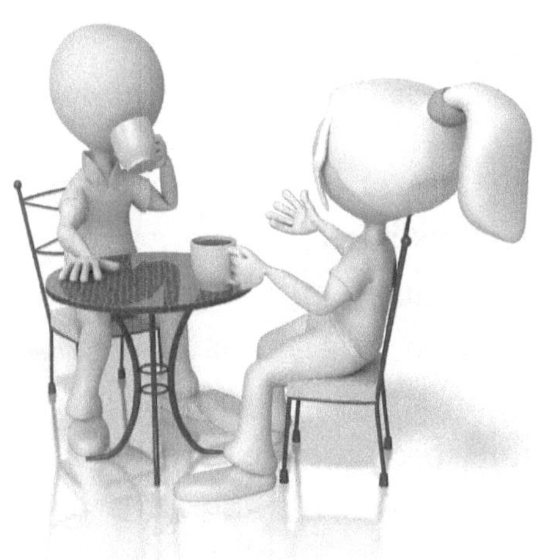

Who to Tell

When talking to others about your MS diagnosis, keep in mind that everyone is unique and has a different personal relationship with you. Some may ask lots of questions and require more answers. Some may accept what you share without questions, while others may say nothing at all and you'll wonder if they even heard, but each will react in their own way to the information you share. Consider each person and their "need to know" status in their relationship with you. The whole world doesn't need to know, but your spouse, children, parents, other family members or close friends may also be affected by how MS affects you, and you may want to let them know.

Before disclosing your diagnosis to employers and co-workers, make sure you assess the pros and cons of sharing your diagnosis in your particular work environment; understand your rights as an employee, and do your homework. You may contact the National MS Society if you're unsure how or if you should address it. The following link from the National MS Society website offers excellent information regarding disclosure decisions: https://www.nationalmssociety.org/Living-Well-With-MS/Work-and-Home/Employment/Disclosure-Decisions

My own decision not to disclose my physical struggles to my employer was based on my personal preference. Had I known I had MS at the time that I resigned, my story may have taken a different turn. As in any work environment, my workplace was undergoing some normal growth changes, which inevitably brought on the expected added stress. During that time, I was dealing with frequent debilitating symptoms, and this time around, the stress only exacerbated them. As someone who wore multiple hats in the work place, my position demanded me to be "on" at all times. However, unbeknownst to me, MS was waging war with me. I loved my job and respected my employers, but not knowing the cause of my struggles, I was unsure how to broach the subject.

I have always put pressure on myself to be the best I can be at whatever I do, so to be fair, I seriously assessed if my job was still a good fit for both myself and my employers. I believe that God has a way of using circumstances to guide us into our next phase of life, and before long, I knew the answer. I submitted a letter of resignation offering to stay on as long as it took to find and/or train my replacement. After all the years I'd invested in the company, it was important to me to leave on good terms, and I did. In retrospect, I see that RRMS, with its characteristic "on again/off again" symptoms, conflicted with my own work ethic in a full-time job. There was no time for being "off" in the role I filled at work. I have no regrets for my decision to resign from a well-paying job that I loved. Given what I knew at the time, it was the right one.

What to Tell

This is my own opinion, but I think that "less is more" in most cases. Outside of the people closest to me, I share only on a "need to know" basis. There are great pamphlets and materials published by MS specific organizations that provide general information to share with others as the situation fits.

http://www.nationalmssociety.org/Resources-Support/Library-Education-Programs/Brochures

Why Tell Anyone at All?

Whether you are someone with a busy family life and young children, an individual with a high-pressure job, or someone with a disability that deals with some degree of limitations, it can be exasperating when others don't understand or decide for you whether you can or cannot do something. I imagine it must be a challenge for those who love us too. Your loved ones may want to "protect" or guard from overloading you, and in so doing, they lovingly back off for fear of overtaxing or exhausting you. Until everyone can openly discuss MS and its side effects, the potential exists for miscommunication, but it doesn't have to be that way if you tell those closest to you how MS affects you.

If the people in your life that matter most understand MS, they will likely not only accept the decisions and adjustments you must make for your life, but they will also be there to provide the support you may need now and in the future. In all fairness, remember that those who are close to you are also affected by how MS affects you. Don't leave them out, leave them wondering, or set yourself up to be misunderstood. You all need one another, and keeping the dialogue open is important.

How to Tell Others

When educating others, share literature if that is helpful. If you decide it's best to tell others at work, in your church or other social situations, let them know you're telling them because you want them to understand how MS affects you (and that MS is not a death sentence.)

For me, the piecing together of this journal was the beginning of my attempt to tell my family how MS was affecting me. I was forced to do *lots* of research. In the process, I saw how completely "MS normal" I am.

The speech/language pathologist that worked with me discussed the importance of *not allowing any disability to dictate our social lives.* I had shared with her the challenge I had participating in conversations while having lunch with the women's group I met with on occasion. I had considered not attending these lunches as I felt "lost" and "spaced out" when several conversations were going on at the same time. She asked me if they knew I had MS. When I told her no, she was genuinely surprised and asked me why. I had lots of reasons (to name just a few):

- I didn't know how to explain it in a sentence or two.
- I didn't want to draw attention to myself.
- It's awkward to talk about it.
- I certainly didn't want to change the subject and make it about me.
- Even explaining it, I feared I would lose my chain of thought (being anxious or nervous can intensify cognitive difficulties.)

Encouraging me to practice summarizing MS in a few sentences so that, when appropriate, I could explain it to others, she had me practice on her. It was *so difficult* to do! However, I'm glad she pushed me, because I needed to be pushed on this topic, and it may be true that you do too. There are certain people in your life you *should* tell, because *you* would want to know if the shoe was on the other foot with someone you care about.

- Don't be surprised when others dismiss your symptoms by telling you all about theirs. It's just how we humans are.
- Don't be offended when others minimize your struggle and suggest you take an aspirin. Forgive them. They just can't understand.
- Don't be discouraged when well-meaning friends give you a book about eating kale to cure your illness or "educate" you on how the poison in your mattress or the hair dye you used twenty years ago might be the cause of your MS. They don't live in your body and can't know how you feel. They have never been forced to be a student of multiple sclerosis. They really do mean well.
- Don't be hurt if others think you're "making something out of nothing," or if they think all the diseases of the world must be due to some sin in your life. They've probably never been blessed with a malady that creates compassion and empathy within us.
- Don't be put out when someone asks how you are, but they don't *really* want to know. Just say "fine."
- Don't become isolated or let MS stop you from enjoying life and time with friends and family.
- Don't be silent when you need to ask for help from time to time. People around us are not mind readers and can't feel what we experience, so when you need help, say it.

So then, how do we communicate to others that this is a central nervous system malfunction or that there are unpredictable "hiccups" or downright *misfires* in the transfer of messages from our brain to the rest of our body? Under my speech pathologist's guidance, I practiced summarizing MS in a few sentences, in my own words and in my own way saying something like this:

> "May I take a minute to explain something that will help us both get the most out of our time together? You may not know this, but I have multiple sclerosis. MS is an immune mediated disease that affects the central nervous system and can affect my balance, cognition, or cause other symptoms that can sometimes be a bit awkward if those around me don't understand it. I am actually a healthy person—I just have MS. I wanted to let you know so that if I get a 'deer in the headlight' look on my face while you're talking or lose my balance or ask for a hand when needed, you'll know that I just had a 'misfire.'"

It doesn't matter how you say it, but if you're anything like me, you may struggle with how to summarize something that affects you to some degree nearly every day of your life.

Okay, now, repeat after me ... *"Hiding, fear, or isolation is never the answer."*

CHAPTER TEN

HIDING, FEAR, AND ISOLATION

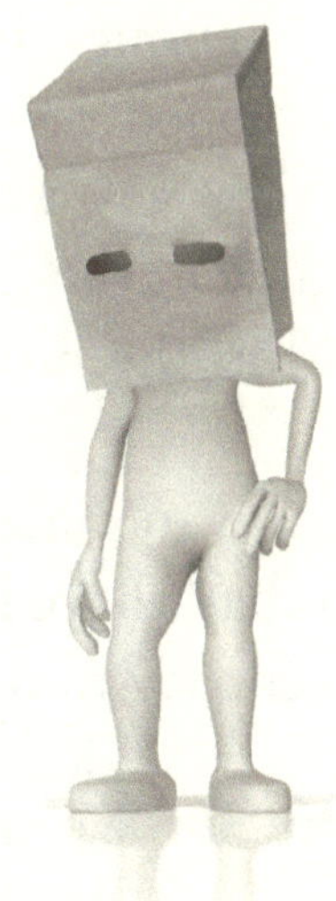

Because MS manifests with a multitude of symptoms, we often struggle with explaining the intensity at which this disease can affect us. We may discover that our confidence has faded, and it's not uncommon to feel frustrated, isolated, or at risk for becoming reclusive. *Isolation is a common reaction when we feel others may not understand.*

Even several years *after* I was diagnosed with MS, "hiding" remained my coping tactic, but take it from me, that approach is *not* effective. I have learned that evading and avoiding when affected by symptoms is a common reaction with many people with MS or other disabilities. The tendency is that if we can't hide symptoms, we hide ourselves by being reclusive. While I may not have mastered how to tell someone how I am affected by MS, sharing the initial manuscript of this book with those close to me was a start. It was my clumsy way to open myself up and allow others into my private world of MS. Some people can just *say* it. Some are affected severely enough by MS that there is no hiding it—it's out in the open or seen through a wheelchair. However, for me, for whatever reason, I struggled with talking about it. I didn't even know how to approach the topic. I felt awkward in the process of coming out of my shell on this topic.

Based on feedback and interactions with others with MS, these are the points that I have found that I and many others with MS want to convey to others:

- MS doesn't define us. We are who we are; we just happen to have MS.
- Don't feel you must ask how we're doing every time you see us, but *thank you for caring.*
- Though MS affects many of us in some way nearly every day (whether in remission or not), we really don't even think about it! There's so much to do and see and enjoy—having MS doesn't change that.

- If you want to help, do so by allowing us to make our own decisions about whether we can or cannot do something. Most of the time, we know our own capabilities, and we won't knowingly take on something we don't think we can handle. We know you love and care about us. We usually know when we're feeling "off" or in relapse. Let us be the judge of our decisions—we'll make mistakes and learn from them.

- Forgive us if we must change our mind at the last minute because our bodies decided not to agree with our will.

- We promise to never take advantage of you or use MS as an excuse *ever*.

- Many times, we just plain hurt. Many of us have lived with neuropathic pain and have survived it long before we knew MS was the culprit, so just because we now know the cause doesn't change a thing. The only difference is that *now YOU know about it, too.* Personally, I'm done hiding.

- I won't answer for others, but as for me, I will seldom say "I can't" when it comes to hanging out with my grandchildren, family or people I love because no matter how I feel, I almost always can, and I certainly always want to. However, I may sometimes need to adjust *what* I do to fit how I'm feeling.

- I have learned that I am a strong woman with a very high tolerance for pain and a very strong will. There may come a time when I have to ask for help, but until then, I will continue to be the stubborn, strong willed woman that God made me and push myself as far as this body and mind will allow.

- Because a varying degree of depression or mood swings is common with MS, we may sometimes feel an "MS cloud" hovering over us. MS can send mixed signals and cause mood swings. We can laugh hysterically over nothing which can easily turn to crying uncontrollably (also over nothing.) Everyone experiences occasional mood swings, but these scrambled emotional responses occur more often in people with MS than in the general public due to the faulty messaging.

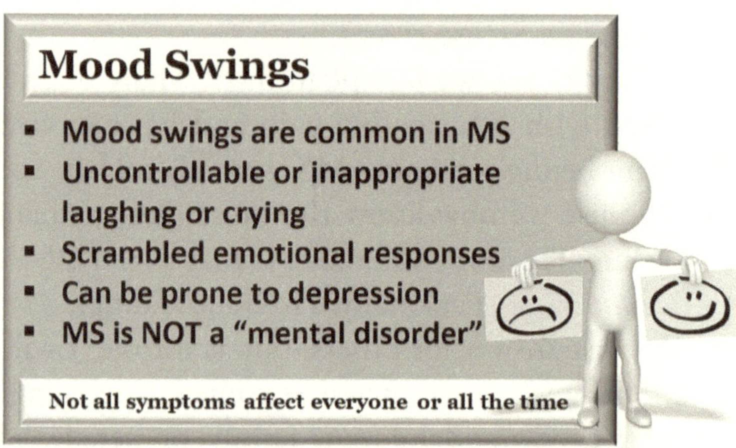

I'll share a more recent experience when my sisters and I took a vacation together. There were hills everywhere, and I must rely on a cane to get up any sized hill. Fully enjoying every minute of the time we had together, I "conquered" one incline after the other and admittedly, I was exhausted; however, I was enjoying the time together and didn't want to be the "wet blanket" among us. Suddenly, silly me burst into tears. I could have been embarrassed, but thankfully I was with my siblings who love and understand me better than anyone. This emotional display was an unexpected MS mood swing likely brought on by fatigue. Thankfully, my sisters didn't act like they felt sorry for me! We have a way of making a joke out of everything, and before long, I was back to laughing, shopping and enjoying the remainder of our day; we just slowed it all down a few notches and allowed more time to rest in between.

MS definitely has its "ups and downs." Just because we burst into tears over nothing from time to time (or start laughing at something we should *not* find funny), doesn't mean we're crazy. It's all part of the complex pathways that occasionally get jumbled up. Sometimes MS is a "barrel of laughs" or a tank of tears!

So, my friend, say it with me: "I'm *not* crazy … I'm *not* crazy … I'm *not* crazy."

There. Doesn't that feel better?

Why We Hide and Become Isolated

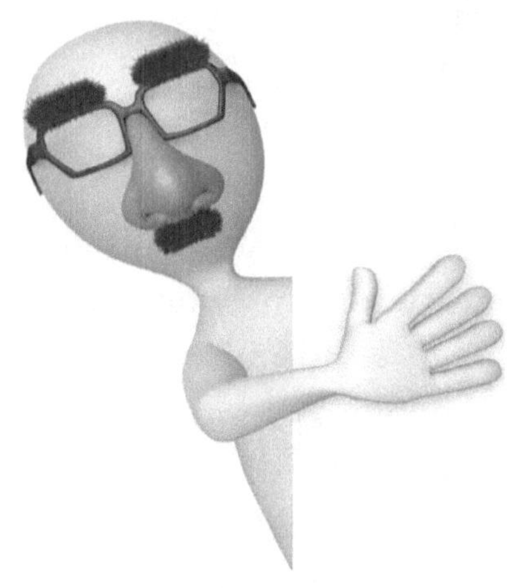

Openly discussing my personal limitations felt like I was asked to stand naked in front of others (UGH!) I had this mistaken mind-set that I always had to "be strong." It was a learning process to grant myself permission to be vulnerable. I'm here to say out loud (or at least in writing) that it's okay to be "imperfect" or weak or weepy or fatigued or clumsy or in pain or an emotional basket case or whatever is popping its ugly little head out today. *It's okay.* Our cognitive, emotional or physical disabilities do not define who we are as individuals.

Bad Habits …

Hiding, fear, and isolation was a bad habit that developed long ago from far too many years being undiagnosed yet dealing with health issues that greatly affected my well-being. In retrospect, I can see how the tendency for isolation and bad coping habits began …

For example:

Within the family, I didn't want to let on that I felt as awful as I did because I didn't know for many years *why* I felt so "off." I had lived with symptoms on and off for so long, it was just part of "life." I thought it would someday go away as insidiously as it had begun. However, as time passed and symptoms worsened without knowing *why* and *what* I had, I hid my symptoms for reasons too numerous (and ridiculous) to mention. This fifteen-year-long "whatever-it-was" was disrupting some aspects of my life, and pain sometimes took its toll on me. Even when I learned I had MS, I still wrestled with old habits of "hiding" and being embarrassed when MS symptoms affected me. Only Dennis knew my struggles, and my secret was safe with him.

Within the work environment, as full-time administrator of a multi-doctor, multi-location practice *and* simultaneously working as VP of operations for its sister consulting company, I was challenged to *always* be on my game. Overseeing over fifty employees in four locations and having leadership roles in two companies (one that required some out-of-state travel), I was wise enough to know I really did need to "fake it" and smart enough to know I could never admit just how much I was struggling with physical pain, jerking movements, balance issues, muscle spasms, and other challenges that were becoming difficult to mask. I allowed myself no room, time, or tolerance for being anything less than efficient. My body, however, disagreed.

Sporadically for years, sharp, stabbing and seemingly random jolts of pain in my face, eye, jaw, limbs, hands, feet (or anywhere, actually) made me "yelp" out loud. They can still wake me from a sound sleep and keep me awake. These indiscriminate, intermittent stabs occur randomly; however, being up and about with daily routines and distractions make them more tolerable during the day than when trying to sit still at work, in a meeting, in church or when trying to sleep. I really didn't know how else to address the symptoms but to recluse when they were present.

It was difficult to explain to *myself* how I was feeling and much more difficult to share it with others. Pain is exhausting, and taking medications for pain was not and is still not an option for me. I'd had my fill of medications when seizures were a regular part of my life, so I did (and do) all I can to deal with pain without prescriptions. Sometimes, it seemed that how I felt physically reflected on how I appeared outwardly, and it was easier to isolate the inner "troll" I often felt I'd become, so I dealt with it the only way I knew—pretending all was well even though I *knew* it wasn't.

Faking It

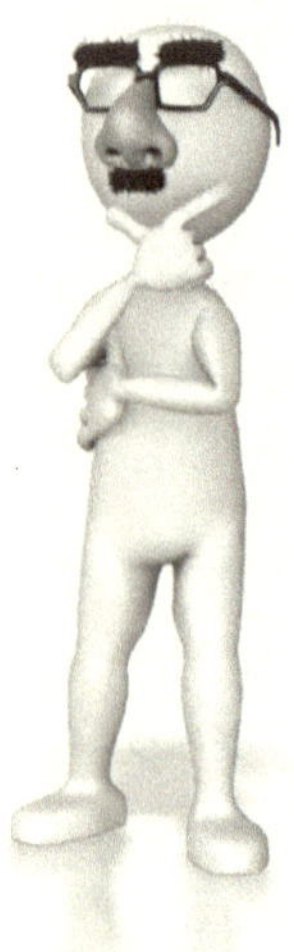

Here is how "faking it" works its way into our lives:

Because we can go for long periods of time feeling very "normal" (in remission), we rightfully keep how we're feeling to ourselves so we don't sound like we're complaining. Then there are the relapses and flare ups when messages to and from our brain, optic nerve and spinal column get confused, and that's when "all hell can break loose."

Indiscriminate MS symptoms have the potential of negatively affecting us not just physically, but socially too. Others may not know, for example, how those with swallowing issues must plan each bite, chew carefully, not talk and eat or laugh and chew or chuckle and breathe at the same time. No one wants to witness food making its way out of our nostrils!

We may have accepted invitations to join others for an evening out. Looking forward to the event, there was no way we could foretell that the illusive MS "ghost" would have a mind of its own. Instead of enjoying an evening out, we may find ourselves barely able to function, or unable to ignore the random shooting neuropathic pain, or drowning in that inexplicable MS fatigue. Because we are hesitant to explain it, we simply don't talk about it. Because we don't talk about it, we set ourselves up for being misunderstood. Because we feel misunderstood, we find ourselves pulling back, and so continues the non-intentional, self-inflicted isolation process.

Somehow, I thought "pretending everything is okay" would make problems disappear. Well, it doesn't. And without an alternate plan, the tendency was to withdraw from socializing because I never knew how I was going to feel. It all sounds so silly when I read this out loud, but if this book is about sharing honest experiences, then let the truth be told. For me, it was easier to withdraw than to face my greatest fear: exposing my struggles or being misunderstood.

What a racket! I really needed to kick the hell out of those bad habits and start anew.

Shut Up!

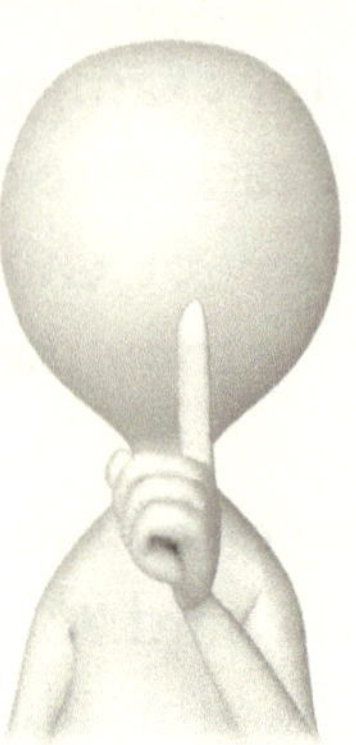

Once I developed a long-standing relationship with being reclusive and "faking it" when symptoms (or relapse) overtook me, I lost sight of the fact that there was another way to approach this. I had spent *so* many years in the workplace and at doctors' visits undiagnosed and wondering, "WHAT IS WRONG WITH ME?" that pulling back and hiding out was the only coping mechanism in my arsenal.

Shut up. Say nothing. Hide. Pretend.

And most of all, don't ever appear to be weak. That is unsightly.

Before I was diagnosed, I kept thinking that this mess would get better if I just identified the cause. Not so.

After I was finally diagnosed, I recognized within myself that I had to shed some bad response habits. For example, because I was sure that others didn't know much (or anything) about multiple sclerosis, I didn't want to sound like I was complaining to tell them how much I was struggling. I didn't want others to think I was "making something out of nothing," so I just said nothing. Because I hate being misunderstood and felt that others may not grasp why I had to back out of a commitment at the last minute (or not commit at all), I continued to "recluse." None of these reactions were purposeful; they were simply how I handled *not* knowing what to do. Admittedly, I'm a born "people pleaser," but I needed to stop caring about what others "might" be thinking, and I needed to rethink how I was thinking. If that sounds confusing, it's because it was!

But now I *knew* the cause and why the messages in my brain were misfiring. Being undiagnosed for *so long* had taken its toll on my emotions and self-image. I had fallen into a decade's long response trap and finally realized I had a great need to rethink this disease and stop pretending I was "fine" all the time. I wasn't fine, and I knew it. But how do I get myself out of this I-need-to-appear-strong mindset? I still had a lot to learn about the nature of this relapsing/remitting disease, and I had a lot to learn about myself! Good heavens; what a mess! I needed an overhaul, and thankfully, the good Lord is in the overhauling business.

Once I had an explanation for all the symptoms I'd been dealing with and I understood more about relapsing-remitting multiple sclerosis, I was empowered to rethink this ordeal and by the grace of God make changes within myself, but until then, I felt I had been fighting two ghostly giants—multiple sclerosis and me! I needed to allow myself to be vulnerable and "imperfect," so I set off on a journey to do a better job facing the truth about myself.

Fear … What a Waste!

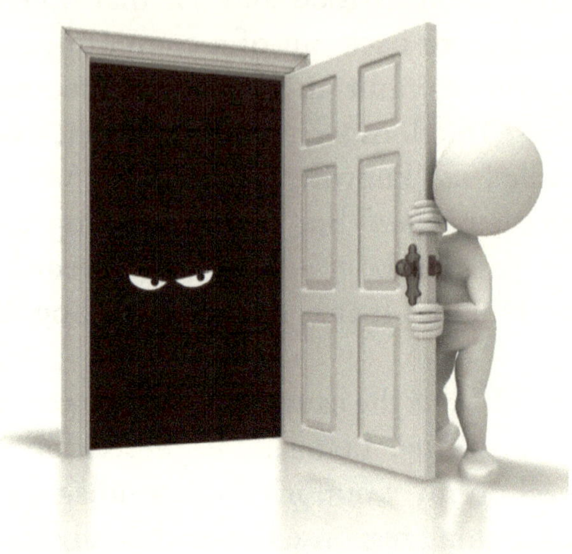

It took me a while to reverse the bad habits of response I had developed over time. Fifteen years of undiagnosed MS, I had inadvertently adopted some ridiculous (but understandable) "fears."

I feared no one would invite me anywhere if they knew how awful I felt.

I feared my kids wouldn't ask me to babysit because they'd think I couldn't handle it.

I feared choking in public or losing bladder control or being unable to follow conversations or getting lost while driving somewhere.

I was struggling not *just* with MS and all the symptoms that accompany it but also with how I fit into the scheme of things. How does one explain something that one doesn't understand or has a difficult time admitting to oneself or talking about with others? *What?* Tell them how I *really* feel?

In my head, I "tried on" all sorts of ways of explaining it …

I thought about this response: "Look, guys, I have MS. I know it will look like I blame everything on MS, but quite frankly, while I do *often* feel really well and actually quite "normal," there are also these unpredictable and frequent periods of utter fatigue, loss of balance, or a debilitating inability to hold a conversation without losing my chain of thought or recall what I or you *just* said *as* I or you were saying it."

And this: "Your mouth is moving, and I know you're speaking English, but I can't for the life of me comprehend what you're saying? I'm aware that I *should* comprehend it, and I'm aware that I can't comprehend it, and I wish I'd have never put myself in this situation in the first place. I feel stupid and confused and 'troll-ish.'"

Or this: "Oh, by the way, while we're on the subject, though I know it sounds like another lame excuse, the truth is that the nerve signals to my brain have gone bonkers sending off-the-wall messages and sensations of being *extremely* hot when there is no logical explanation for it. So while you're sitting here in your cozy little sweater in a seventy-two-degree environment, I'm dressed down as much as much as I dare and feeling like I'll distract or draw attention to myself if I try to sneak out of the room for relief from the inward burning that is even more intense than a menopausal hot flash! I'm *so* inexplicably hot that it is nearly impossible to sit comfortably when I feel like internal combustion is imminent."

Or how about this: "While we're sitting here chatting, I'm trying my best to hide the shooting, stabbing, burning pain searing through my arms or legs or feet or hands or jaw or eye or face or maybe tonight it's just that annoying, distracting itching/tingling sensation that's driving me *nuts*, and I'm *so* miserable that being 'with it' right now is *really* difficult … but if I tell you any of this, you might think I'm *always* this way when I'm not."

Itching Sensations

- Neurologically induced (dysesthesias)
- Distracting, annoying itch for no apparent reason
- "Creepy-crawly" "pins-&-needles" sensation
- Can be felt anywhere on body including inner ear, fingers, toes, face, nose, lips, etc.
- Feels like a rash starting, but there's nothing there

Not all symptoms affect everyone or all the time

Even more perplexing is that these various symptoms and sensations can come and go; disappear forever, stay for months or weeks, or maybe never go away. Toss a little MS mood swing in the mix and we have a perplexing mess nicely wrapped in a nut bag, therefore, I deemed it easier to just shut up and withdraw. But really, in the big picture, it *wasn't* easier. It is in this way that I ended up retreating, hiding, and isolating myself.

If you are anything like I was, at some point, we must step back and reevaluate these old habits that developed unintentionally over time and ask ourselves, "Is there a better way to handle this?" We need to get our footing, find our place, acknowledge how this disease may have affected us emotionally, socially and psychologically, then make the determination to move forward and *not* allow MS to define us. For me, holding fast to my faith in Jesus Christ, my Higher Power, has been my springboard for everything positive and the source from which I drew my strength to get on the right track in dealing with MS.

At some point, those of us who fell into bad habits from too many years of being undiagnosed (or too many years allowing MS to dictate our "now" or our future, or whatever particular hang up we may have) need to reevaluate ourselves and the direction of our lives, establish goals going forward, and most importantly, *claim the freedom God gave us to live our lives to its fullest.* Life is far too magnificent to get stuck along the way.

Whether MS, its symptoms, our emotional, social, or physical well-being is challenging, manageable, or somewhere in between, we benefit greatly to aspire to get the most out of life, and therefore, if we've not done so already, it's high time to kick the habit of bad habits!

CHAPTER ELEVEN

ODYSSEY TO DIAGNOSIS

There are valid reasons why diagnosing multiple sclerosis can be a long and somewhat frustrating ordeal. MS symptoms are often random and varied, and there is a multitude of nerve impulses and "connections" that can go awry and affect the central nervous system making it nearly impossible to identify, especially at its first symptoms. It's not unusual for diagnosis to take years, as it is clouded by the disease's apparent randomness and symptoms which mimic other maladies. Patients with undiagnosed MS can become frustrated, and often, they just stop bringing up symptoms to their doctors.

Overworked, time-constrained physicians don't have time to hear years of symptoms; some don't listen or take patient complaints seriously. However, I believe most physicians and specialists *do* care and do all they know to get to the root of the problem. They are constrained in a system that deprives them of the time that they genuinely want to give each patient. Imagine yourself having to piece together a very large puzzle without seeing the picture on the box.

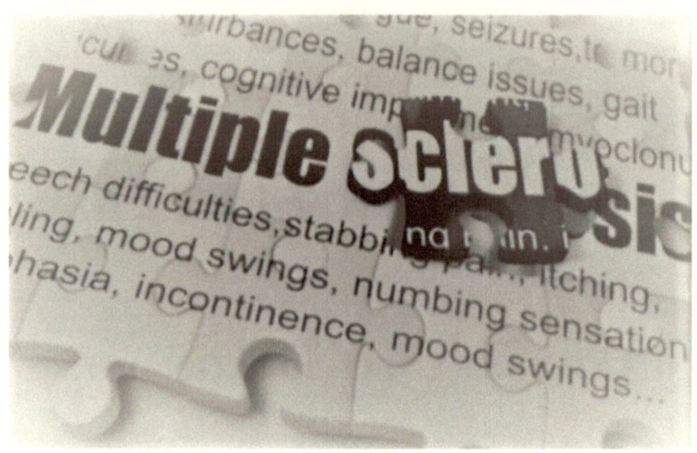

You don't know what it is that you're supposed to be piecing together. MS is like that jigsaw puzzle, only the pieces are not all present for many years. We can't blame doctors for that! Yet until diagnosed, patients are left to fend for themselves to get the bottom of a disease that relapses and remits without warning and with fluctuating symptoms and often over a period of years.

Is There an Absolute Test for MS?

Currently, there is no single laboratory test that can conclusively identify MS, nor is there any one test that can absolutely rule it out, so we certainly can't fault doctors for not knowing a patient has MS. According to the National Institute of Health, "MS can be among the most difficult of all diseases to diagnose because of the bewildering number of symptoms it causes and the multiple ways in which they can present … The diagnosis may be especially difficult, or indeed impossible, when the patient is older, when symptoms are strictly progressive, or when there has been only one episode of neurologic dysfunction ..."[xviii]

While an MRI is extremely useful in detecting central nervous system demyelination and is a valuable tool in determining a more definitive diagnosis of MS, lesions or scarring are not always evident on an MRI. According to the National MS Society, about five percent of people who have "clinically-definite MS" may initially show no lesions on an MRI because of "silent areas of the brain that don't produce symptoms." They also state "it is not always possible to make a specific correlation between what is seen on the MRI scan and the person's clinical signs and symptoms."[xix]

Specialists ...

Like a car with mechanical issues, the journey to diagnosis can be expensive, frustrating, and feel as if it is one dead end after the other. Here is an analogy Dennis shared with me that elaborates the point quite well.

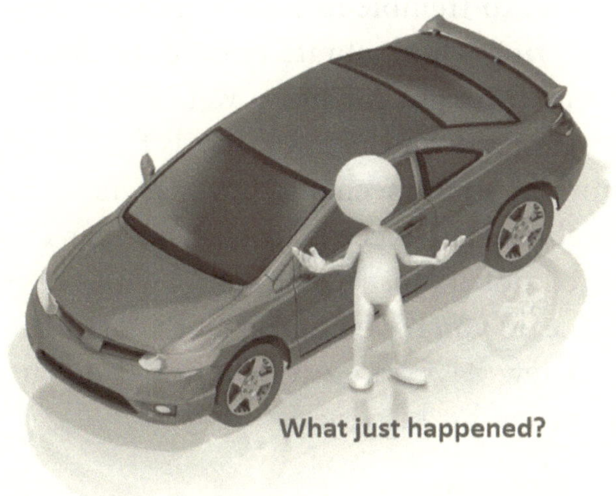

It's a beautiful sunny day, and you decide to take a ride and enjoy a leisurely drive through the countryside. Suddenly, the car starts shaking violently and makes a loud, squealing sound. A strong vibration in the steering wheel forces you to fight the wheel in order to drive to the side of the road. Your heart is racing and you shout to no one in particular, "What just happened?" You are baffled as you wonder what's wrong with your car. Is it your brakes? Do you have a flat tire? Are you low on oil? (Not that you've ever checked the oil ever in your life.) Did the tie rods suddenly break loose from the car and now lay in the middle of the road? You're unsure what a tie rod is, but you bet it's important for your car to function properly.

At this point, you are fearful to drive another mile. You arrange for your car to be towed to the nearest garage. On the way there, the mechanic asks you how the car was acting. "Well, all seemed normal as I drove the speed limit, but all of a sudden, the car made a loud noise that sounded like a medley of cats fighting and angry, hungry babies! Then it began to tremble like my pet boxer after his bath, then the steering wheel vibrated like an off balanced washing machine. It fought me like a wet cat and forced me to pull over to the side of the road. It was frightening!"

"Hmmm," the mechanic says as he scratches his unshaven chin. He proceeds to tell you that it will cost a few hundred dollars just to look at it with no guarantees. What choice do you have but to pay the man and hope for the best? A few days and a few hundred dollars later the mechanic makes his big reveal.

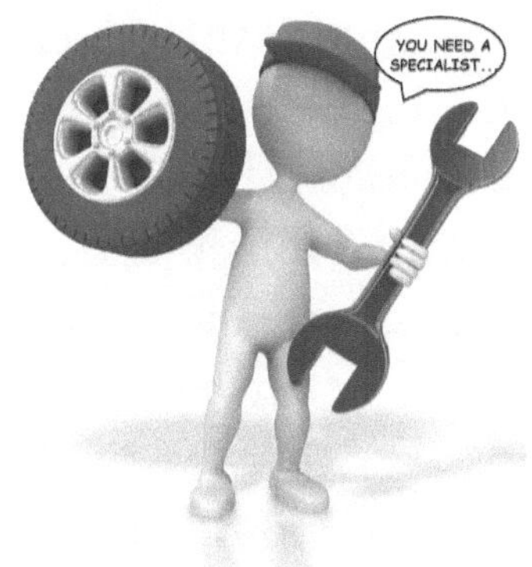

"Sorry, Ma'am, but I couldn't find anything wrong with your car. Are you *sure* it made those funny noises? Maybe you ran over a rock or hit a pothole? That would explain the shaking and vibration. Could you have run over a squirrel? That could explain the screeching noises. If I were you I'd have it towed over to a transmission specialist who might be able to find a problem." So off to the transmission specialist it's towed. The "specialist" questions you about the noise and shaking; he examines the car and runs more diagnostic tests then charges two hundred more dollars to look at it. Several days later he lets you know he couldn't find the problem and recommends a mechanic that specializes in radiators.

The radiator specialist finds nothing wrong and tells you so, but he too must charge you for his time and "expertise." He recommends an electrical expert that will run more diagnostics on your charging system: battery, alternator, starter, wiring—the works! After many exhaustive tests, he suggests that all these problems may just be "in your head." And with that, he hands you his three-hundred-dollar bill.

Does this all sound familiar?

Generally, if patients visit their doctors because they are having, for example, double vision, their doctor may refer them to an ophthalmologist. If patients are having bladder issues, they may be treated for a bladder infection. If they're experiencing balance issues, referral to the ear, nose, and throat specialists might be on the agenda. Whether or not a patient is diagnosed with MS, rightfully and typically, doctors will order lab tests to rule out infection or disease. However, when tests return within normal limits, doctors may scratch their heads and refer you to a specialist who, after more tests, may also scratch *his* head and let you know he's stumped.

Before one knows they have MS or even after diagnosis, patients often find that doctors tend to treat each symptom as a separate issue, and in some ways, MS symptoms do appear to present separately. To add more challenge to the mix, some symptoms really *can* be separate issues.

Got Ailments?

I have experienced in most doctor visits through the years, that whether the *cause* for certain symptoms was identified or not, I nearly always left that appointment with a prescription of some kind for something. To avoid misunderstanding, I want to make it clear that I am not against prescription medications, and I take several for managing blood pressure and cholesterol; I certainly believe that prescription medications have their place. I do, however, also consider natural alternatives as well.

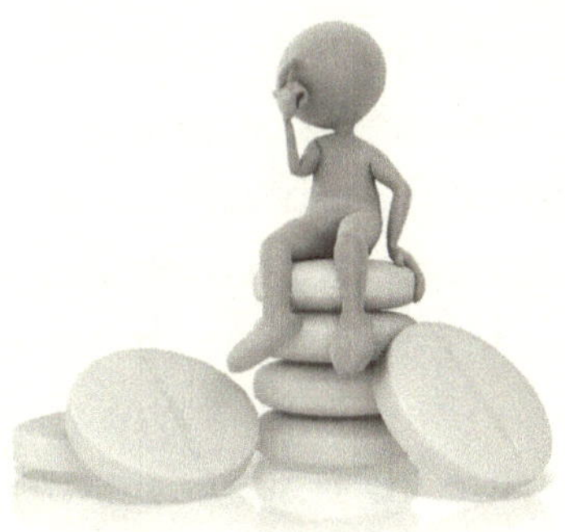

My personal experience with traditional medicine is that medical doctors are often "ready at a sniffle" to write a prescription for whatever ailment we may have.

Got shooting pain in your left eye? *Here's a pain pill.*

Got bladder issues? *Here's an antibiotic or medication to reduce episodes of incontinence.*

Feeling dizzy? *Here's a pill for dizziness.*

Got muscle spasms? *Here's a muscle relaxer.*

Got side effects from the meds your taking? *Here's a prescription for the side effects.*

And if those medications for the side effects bother you, *we've got a pill for that too!*

I can't stress enough how important it is for us to be informed about MS, its symptoms and treatment options to better enable us, along with our doctor(s), to be part of our medical *team*. One thing I have learned about relapsing-remitting multiple sclerosis is how important it is to find a doctor who understands MS or is willing to learn more about it. While problems with vision, bladder control, fatigue, balance, or other issues may be common MS symptoms, there can also be an actual infection or problem that may not be MS related; we don't want to "blame" every symptom on MS, yet we also should be informed enough to know that MS does manifest in a variety of ways.

Our bodies are intricately designed machines, so there are many unknowns and unanswered questions regarding multiple sclerosis. In chatting with others who have had RRMS for decades, there is a surprisingly large number who express hesitation or discouragement in seeking traditional medical treatment for MS. Many complain that they feel "unheard, rushed, or misunderstood." In defense of most doctors, I think they strive to accurately diagnose and treat their patients, but I also think that the medical community is all-too-often uninformed about MS or clinically isolated by their specialty to navigate the MS maze. Traditional doctors' predictable response is to treat individual symptoms with various medications, many of which could have potential side effects that are worse than the disease itself.

An ever-increasing number of people with MS are moving toward a more natural approach for minimizing and treating MS symptoms and relapses. Some of these natural approaches may include, for example, dietary changes ranging from the Paleo diet (https://multiplesclerosisnewstoday.com/living-with-ms/ms-diet-nutrition/paleo-diet-and-ms/), The Wahl's Protocol® (https://terrywahls.com/) or the Swank Diet (http://www.swankmsdiet.org/the-diet/) along with (or in some cases instead of) disease modifying therapy (DMT) rather than relying first, foremost, or only on prescriptions.

In her book *The Wahls Protocol*, Dr. Terry Wahl's (diagnosed in 2000 with MS) writes, "...The names we first put on most chronic diseases are the result of observations made prior to the scientific understanding of the biochemical workings of individual cells. Billions of dollars are spent by the National Institutes of Health and by the drug industry studying disease symptoms and drugs to control those symptoms. By contrast, very little is spent to study how to create optimal health and vitality through life-style choice that can lead to healthier biochemistry and, consequently, healthier people."[xx]

While traditional medical doctors may seldom suggest natural remedies that may help reduce symptoms or minimize relapses, they more often resort to pharmaceuticals first and foremost. In contrast, naturopathic practitioners focus primarily on natural remedies. They have greater limitations on their scope of practice regarding dispensation of prescription medications. In fact, as of the date of this printing, only 18 states and the District of Columbia have licensing or regulation laws for naturopaths.[xxi]

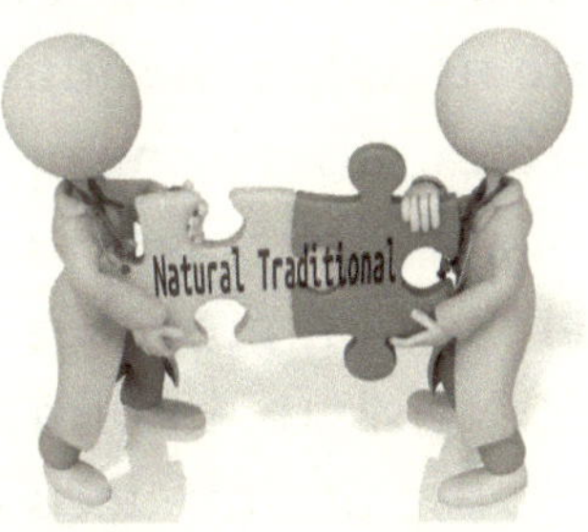

Personally, I prefer a team approach, which allows me the freedom to utilize the valuable knowledge and skill set of both a traditional medical doctor and a naturopathic doctor. The multibillion dollar pharmaceutical industry has a huge influence in the healthcare realm and medical teaching institutions, and they stand to benefit through the sale of pharmaceuticals rather than support the studies and advancement of natural remedies. As the one whose body is impacted by my health decisions, I opt to keep an open dialogue with both my medical doctor and naturopathic professional. Be sure to discuss beforehand any changes you may be considering including dietary, herbal, or vitamin/mineral supplements to ensure that your decisions do not conflict with current medications or have potential negative ramifications you may not have considered.

To date, there is no cure for multiple sclerosis, but there are comfort measures such as therapeutic massage, herbs and essential oils, acupuncture, chiropractic treatment, or alternatives such as yoga, Pilates, Tai Chi and other options that may offer relief of symptoms for many with MS. You may not often hear these recommendations from your family doctor or neurologist; they are not usually trained in this school of thought and some may not view these as legitimate alternatives. Some practitioners may give us an eye rolling or lecture us about the "unscientific, unproven nature of these remedies" if we bring up alternative/adjunct therapies or naturopathy. However, despite the tendency for some traditional medical providers to "poo poo" alternative medicine, it's wise to inform your primary-care physician or neurologist of any decisions to incorporate adjunct therapy in your course of treatment—especially if you are taking prescription medications or have certain health issues that should be considered in your decision. I have a wonderful family physician and renal specialist that *do* listen and *do* respect my input, and I rely on them to advise if there is a safety reason I may not have considered.

My personal decisions or how I choose to deal with MS is an ever-learning process. No one knows more than the person living in his or her body how best to measure symptoms or determine if they are manageable at any given time in our personal journey with MS. Some choose not to take any medications, steroids or injections; some take whatever is recommended without question. It is our right and our responsibility to do what we feel is best in our individual situations. I am always cautious when taking either natural supplements or prescription medications.

While the decisions that I make may not be right for you and may change as I discover new ways to deal with MS, I want to emphasize that we should never hesitate to talk openly with our medical team about any ideas or concerns that we may have. I have had far too many reactions to prescription medications that sent me to Urgent Care or the ER. My best advice is to *do your homework*. Base your decisions on knowledge, on what works for you, on your open dialogue with your medical team, and on whether the side effects of any medication outweigh the symptoms of MS. It's your body. It's your life. It's your decision.

CHAPTER TWELVE

RELAPSE HAS A MIND OF ITS OWN

It's not unusual to feel so good for so long, that someone with RRMS can forget they even have this disease at all. Except for the "usual" symptoms to which we've learned to adjust, life can be flowing smoothly and wonderfully with minimal to no symptoms for months when, seemingly out of nowhere, relapse hits without warning.

When the central nervous system (CNS) becomes inflamed, it can cause more damage to the myelin sheath and nerves resulting in the disturbance or interruption to nerve impulses. Exacerbation of symptoms is consequential, varying from person to person or relapse to relapse (depending on the extent or location of the attack). Relapse can interfere with mobility, function, strength, balance, vision, or a list of other things. An unwelcomed guest that pops in unannounced, relapse can steal our energy and time, linger far longer than expected, create a mess when present, doesn't care if we're exhausted by its presence, then skedaddle only when good and ready (if at all).

Relapse has a mind of its own!

Flare-Ups

Depending on the type of MS or other factors (such as whether a disease modifying therapy [DMT], special diet, or natural remedy is effective or not), relapse can be short-lived with minor symptoms, or lasting without remission of symptoms. It may take years to figure out what sparks a relapse for each individual. Knowing our triggers can sometimes help us dodge a flare-up, but there can be a wide variety of triggers that elicit a relapse one time and not every time or ever again.

Common causes of flare-ups can be infections or illness, overexertion, stress, or even a reaction to vaccines or medications. Keep in mind that not every symptom experienced is related to MS. Sometimes there may be a completely unrelated issue going on that should not be ignored and may need medical attention.

If you choose to use DMTs to keep relapses at bay, the MSAA (Multiple Sclerosis Association of America) provides a helpful program for determining if a treatment is right for you and encourages patients to "take an active, decision-making role in selecting a treatment." The MSAA explains that there are "an extraordinary number of factors (that) need to be considered when choosing an appropriate MS therapy or switching from one DMT to another. Among the numerous questions to consider include: What are the therapies? Am I a candidate? What should I know about each one? How will my body react to taking one of these medications? How are the different medications administered? What about the costs or insurance? Once I have begun taking a DMT, how do I know if the one I am prescribed is working?"[xxii]

One Hot Chick

I have learned that being physically ill is a definite trigger for me. For example, in 2015, I had pneumonia that crept up on me unexpectedly following what I thought was just a bad cold. My sister-in-law drove me to the doctor's office because I'd had fever of 103° since the day before and a tight, unrelenting cough. By the time I got to my appointment, my temperature was 104°. I must have looked like a ragamuffin, as the nurse brought me ice water and put an ice pack on the back of my neck. My doctor listened to my lungs, took X-rays, told me I had pneumonia and called in a few prescriptions to fight infection.

By 2:00 a.m., Dennis woke me in a panic.

"Jeanne, your temperature is 106°! What should I do?" he asked desperately.

"Help me take a tepid shower," I weakly instructed.

I was shivering uncontrollably, but the shower successfully lowered my temperature to 102°; low enough to get me through the night. I was back to the doctor's office the next morning where the nurse practitioner gave me a gentle "scolding" for not seeking medical attention with a fever that high. I replied, "A trip to the ER would have meant sitting in the waiting area with a 106° temperature for who knows how long before *they* put me in a tepid shower to lower my temperature." She smiled and nodded in agreement.

All said, I got over the pneumonia just fine, but an MS relapse *kicked my butt* for several months following that illness. This incident was my first clear awareness that illness can send someone with MS into relapse—myself included!

Take That!

In April of 2016, I had what the ER doctor recorded as an anaphylactic reaction to a blood pressure medication I had taken for years. As seen in the before/after photos below, my face, arms, and neck were like one huge hive. I felt my throat begin to tighten and knew it was time to take action and go to the ER.

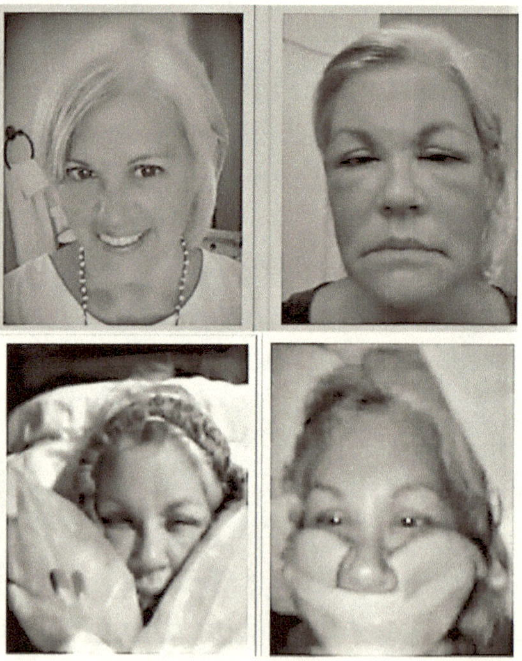

In addition to an injection and a take-home prescription, I applied icepacks and essential oils to calm down the itching, swelling, and burning reaction. I even tried refrigerated banana peels (don't laugh, I was desperate.) It took nearly two weeks of burning, stinging, and swelling before I no longer showed a physical reaction to my medication, but worse than the allergic reaction was the full-blown relapse that followed intermittently for months.

W-w-what's Ha-ha-happening?

Over the following weeks, I had increased stuttering, what I call "cognitive hiccups," and unrelenting muscle spasms and twitches that were not just annoying, but some were downright painful. One muscle spasm twisted my foot sideways and lasted over four hours, keeping me up most of the night and leaving me with a sprained and swollen ankle on which I was unable to walk for several days.

In an effort to find blood pressure–lowering medication to replace the one to which I had an allergic reaction, my doctor prescribed multiple and various medications to find one that would work. My blood pressure had now gotten dangerously out of control, and from April through November of that year, my doctor and I battled this body rebellion unsuccessfully while my blood pressure spiked into hypertensive crisis. At a loss for options, he referred me to a renal specialist who prescribed a combination of medications that finally brought the BP under control. Warned in advance that the new medication had side effects that would likely resolve after several weeks, I was told, "You're probably going to hate me, and I encourage you to call the office as often as you need to, but just be warned that this med usually works, but you're probably going to feel like crap while you adjust." (Yes, he really said that!)

At first, the medication made me feel like a blithering drunk. Water retention caused my feet and ankles to be unrecognizable as my own, and it induced *extreme* fatigue and other reactions before finally adjusting.

So What?

I tell this part of my story not because the elevated blood pressure issue or negative reaction to medications were part of MS, but *because of these issues*, I went into another full-blown, months-long relapse from which I never fully recovered. Stuttering, loss of balance, and cognitive issues increased as did leg cramps, tics, tingling, and other sensations and symptoms.

Muscle Spasms/Spasticity

- Involuntary kicking or muscle twitching
- Frequent or constant "charlie horse" in leg(s), rib cage or any muscle group
- Spasms (short-lived or lasts for hours)
- Spasticity (continuous contraction, stiffness, tightness of muscle groups)
- Muscle fatigue makes spasms worse

Not all symptoms affect everyone or all the time

There wasn't much I knew to do at the time to prevent the MS relapse following this allergic reaction, but there are many things I *can* do to help prevent MS flare-ups as much as possible. Knowing my limits and living within them, taking extra precautions during flu season, eating right and getting enough exercise to keep me healthy without overdoing it is a start.

It's important to be proactive in keeping healthy with MS. Something as simple as a cold or flu, stress, or even a bladder infection can trigger a flare-up or ignite a relapse. Getting a good night's rest is important as well, and sometimes that's almost impossible when muscle spasms and pain keep us up or wake us from a sound sleep. Not all symptoms are directly MS related. It's a good idea to talk to your pharmacist to help you determine if any medication you are taking may have sleep disrupting side effects.

When in relapse, we often experience more fatigue than usual and would do well to give ourselves permission to take it easy and get as much rest as possible. Relapse can also cause even more heat sensitivity; avoid getting overheated, which can intensify MS symptoms. Recovering from a relapse can take weeks or even months; if there is more nerve damage, some symptoms may not go away fully or may not go away at all.

In her article, "How to Treat and Prevent an MS Flare-Up," Stephanie Watson writes, "With multiple sclerosis (MS), you'll have good days and bad days. You might feel fine for weeks or months, and then your symptoms suddenly get worse. Days when your old symptoms pop up again or new symptoms start are called relapses, attacks, or flare-ups. Everyone's flare-ups are different. Some are mild. Others are severe. The goal is to prevent relapses. When your symptoms do get worse, know how to treat them so you can feel better faster."[xxiii]

It may not be possible to prevent all MS flare-ups, but doing all we can to minimize them is essential. While there is no cure for MS, there are medications available that may help manage MS flare-ups. It is up to each of us to research and decide for ourselves what the best course of treatment is for maintaining as much mobility and reducing as many flare-ups as we can.

There are many disease-modifying drugs that are said to slow the progression of MS or halt a relapse in its tracks. I am not qualified to assess or comment on any of them except to say that there are more than I can wrap my brain around! From interferon injections (i.e., Avonex®, Betaseron®, ExTavia®, Rebif®, etc.) to glatiramer acetate injections (i.e., Copaxone®, Glatopa®, etc.) to intravenous infusions such as Lemtrada®, Novantrone®, Ocrevua™, Tysabri®, etc. and oral medications such as Aubagio®, Gilenya®, Tecfidera™ …the list seems endless and can be overwhelming when you take the time to read the benefits, side effects or warnings.

While I am slow to jump on the prescription band wagon, I have read responses from many that have had positive feedback. However, with common side effects like flu-like symptoms, muscle aches and/or joint pain, chest pain, flushing, fast heartbeat, anxiety, shortness of breath, itching as well as potential long-term effects like liver problems, ongoing nausea, hair loss, diarrhea, etc., it is worth assessing if the long-term benefits outweigh the risks.

When "doing your homework" about the right treatment for you, the MSAA's S.E.A.R.C.H.™ program may be helpful. The acronym stands for Safety, Effectiveness, Access, Risks, Convenience, Health Outcomes. You can see the webinar or read more about it here: https://mymsaa.org/ms-information/search/.

While our personal symptoms with MS may be very manageable with just a few alterations, we still need to confront the giant and initiate addressing where we are in this MS journey. For me, I found it was time to chat with my doctor about the physical challenges with which I was dealing. He recommended physical, occupational, and speech therapy to address the issues that gave me the most challenges. I gladly followed up with these options and was impressed with the knowledge these trained therapists had in dealing with challenges brought on by MS. It was encouraging to find that through these various types of therapy, I was able to see some improvement and benefited from the educational aspect of how to manage symptoms that were likely not going to go away.

CHAPTER THIRTEEN

Confronting the Giant

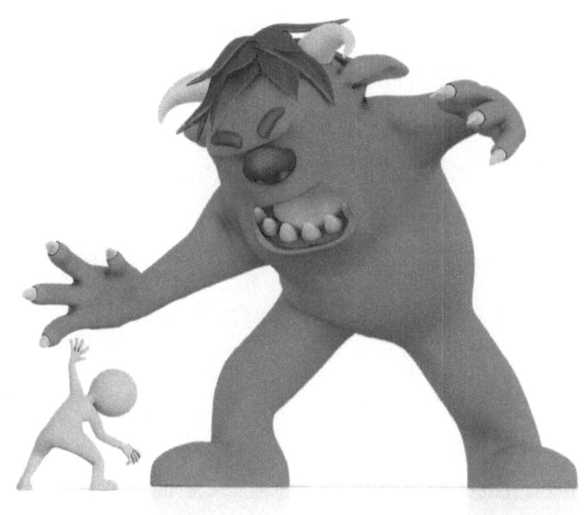

By now, you have probably figured out why it is that people with relapsing-remitting multiple sclerosis write books such as these. Sometimes we just need to sort out some thought patterns that resulted from being uninformed and undiagnosed for too long, and maybe this is why you are reading or sharing this book with someone you love.

MS can be complicated, but it doesn't have to be. It can seem like a giant when you are not aware of how it can affect you, or you don't have a game plan when you *are* affected. Fortunately, there are *many* tools available to help compensate for some "malfunctions"—but they do no good if you don't use them.

Use Your Tools

I remained reluctant to reach out for help through physical, occupational, speech, and adjunct therapies because I felt like I wasn't "disabled enough" to warrant this kind of help. However, after I took advantage of these options to address balance, hand weakness, cognitive, and swallowing challenges, I experienced how these options benefitted me. Be mindful that everyone is different and what works or does not work for one person with MS does not mean others will have the same experience.

Occupational Therapy

Occupational therapy (OT) can help individuals of any age to accomplish the daily activities they need for a more productive life after an injury, illness or disability. I was referred to an occupational therapist to help me improve grip strength. Due to hand weakness, the simple act of pushing a grocery cart, using a manual can opener, lifting an object, or even grasping the bedspread to make the bed in the morning had been a challenge for me for quite some time.

> ## Loss of Grip Strength
>
> - **Impaired hand and dexterity function common in MS**
> - **Hand strength not routinely evaluated in clinical workups**
> - **Reasons vary from numbness, pain, lack of coordination, muscle fatigue, nerve damage**
>
> **Not all symptoms affect everyone or all the time**

The OT helped me understand the physiological aspect of why my hands were weak and instructed me in appropriate hand strengthening exercises. Using one-pound weights, exercise putty, and stretching exercises, in six weeks I went from being unable to close my fist to being able to not only make a fist but have more strength than I had before OT. I have continued to maintain enough strength and flexibility to achieve more tasks than I could previously and have found other ways to accomplish activities of daily living by taking advantage of tools like an electric can opener and gizmos that allow me to open jars with limited strength.

If you're anything like me, you're probably not going to just "accept" a weakness until you've tried everything that may bring positive results. If hand or grip strength is still a challenge, there are countless tools available to fit just about any particular need.

Energy Conservation

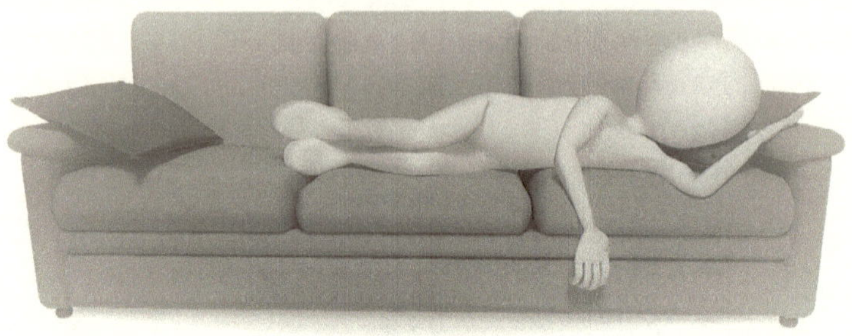

One of the most useful pieces of information I learned during OT was applying the concept of *energy conservation* to my everyday life. Undoubtedly, a trip to the grocery store or running basic errands had me so wiped out that I was useless for the remainder of the day. Now, I am mindful that there is only "so much" energy to spend each day, so I need to be thrifty, use my energy bank efficiently, and not "spend it all in one place."

Working simply and efficiently allows me more independence without being so overwhelmed by fatigue. To implement energy conservation, I now prioritize tasks and plan ahead so I can combine activities, avoid unnecessary steps, and sort tasks so that activities that take the most energy aren't bundled together. I'm at my best in the morning, so the more strenuous tasks are done then. I try to rest as soon as I see I'm wearing out. Frequent short rests go a long way in completing the day's activities. I have learned that when I push myself past my limit, I pay for it for days. The key is to rest *before* I'm worn out. Examples of ways I have applied energy conservation:

I now use online grocery shopping with store-to-car delivery service—a game changer for me. Many large and small chain grocery stores offer this service free, and some offer home delivery if you live within a certain radius of the store. I love the convenience of placing items in the online cart through the week. When we're ready, Dennis or I pay online and select the time range for pick up. The store employee delivers and places the order in my car and voila—energy conservation at work!

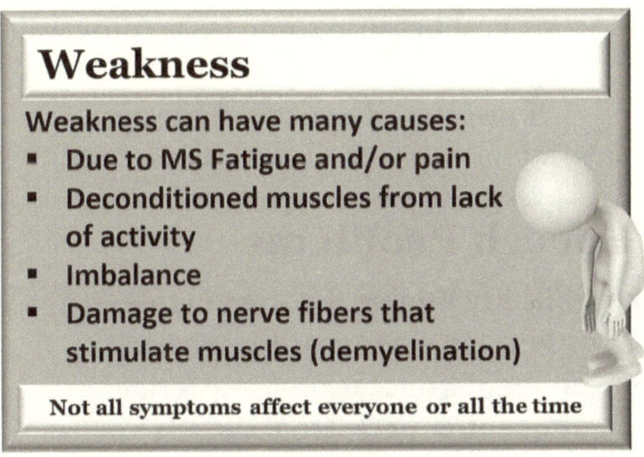

I no longer try to clean my entire house in one day. Instead, I divide home chores, errands away from home and other activities (like bathing the dogs, gardening or cleaning out a closet) into multiple days and do my best to get done early enough to rest before dinner.

After a lifetime of folding laundry while standing near the dryer, I now fold laundry while sitting down. Fortunately for me, Dennis never hesitates to roll up his sleeves and help with whatever is needed.

I will force myself to sit rather than pace when on the phone.

I go into "energy reserve" if I have a lot of activities planned for later in the day. I may read a book (write a book) or keep myself busy with more sedentary activities so that I have the energy I need later in the day.

Applying energy conservation to my daily thought process has made a huge difference, given me some control over fatigue, and made me more productive. Now, there is energy left over for things I want to do. I had to learn that the world won't end because some tasks must wait.

Language/Speech Therapy

A speech pathologist is trained to diagnose, assess, and treat people with communication and swallowing disorders. Patients with MS often deal with challenges ranging from cognitive misfires and memory issues to stuttering or swallowing disorders. I was given a series of exercises to strengthen the muscles used for speech and swallowing and to help with some cognitive issues.

I had already been using technology and other tools to remind me of events or chores and to help with organization of thought, but she also introduced me to apps that exercise the brain and help improve memory. I have been using these daily as well as applying many other strategies.

Like many people with diseases that affect us neurologically, I am *extremely* forgetful; however, by using every tool I can, I *rarely* miss commitments or forget events or appointments, and I maintain my to-do lists and upcoming tasks. These tools may not help me recall what I was just thinking or talking about, but by golly, I won't forget the things my tools help me remember.

Apps, buzzers, beepers, tools, or alarms only work if you use them. It will make your life easier, take out some of the worry of forgetting, and will compensate for a few of the brain cells we may have dropped along the way.

Physical Therapy

Working with individuals who have a disease, injury, or deformity that hinders their activities of daily living, physical therapists are trained to help individuals improve balance, strengthen muscles, find new ways to do things with a disability, or recover from injury. Using alternative measures to surgery or medications or as a post-operative measure to return to normal activities, physical therapy (PT) is worth considering.

I didn't realize how much independence I'd lost due in part to MS's effect on my balance. I found myself constantly assessing if I could accomplish certain tasks when away from home. Walking from my car to the grocery store had me looking for parking places where I could use the cart to keep me upright on my trek to the store. From there, I had the cart as my "crutch." I had done this for several years and didn't realize how much I depended on it for balance.

There were many errands I simply stopped doing because I had nothing on which to rely to help with balance; those errands eventually became tasks I'd save for when Dennis was with me and I could use his arm to keep me balanced. I found ways to adjust to doing what I needed to do, but without realizing it, little by little I had lost a great deal of independence and gained a lot of apprehension for doing many tasks myself. Yet I never thought I was "bad enough" for a cane or assistive device.

My time in physical therapy taught me appropriate exercises to maintain some degree of balance through exercises to strengthen muscles and joints. However, PT was not enough to gain the independence I needed to accomplish the goals without some kind of assistance for balance. When my physical therapist asked if I had ever considered using a cane, I knew it was time to stop pretending that things were going to be as they were once upon a time. She showed me how to use a cane, explained the type of cane I should buy and how to measure for correct length. Even though I knew I needed the assistance, it still took weeks to even start looking for a cane. Silly as it sounds, it was a big step for me. I needed to think this through, give myself permission, and mentally adjust to using one. *I just didn't want to use a cane!* Oh, vain thing that I am!

Walking Difficulties

Gait problems can be due to:

- Nerve damage that effects coordination
- Fatigue or limited endurance
- Compromised balance
- Spasticity / stiffness
- Numbness or Weakness

Not all symptoms affect everyone or all the time

Until someone has walked a mile in our spastic legs or experienced the battle between the will and the central nervous system in rebellion, they have *no* idea what it's like to have to put thought, planning or energy into doing things that we didn't have to think about at all at one time.

For several years, Dennis and I noticed that when I walked on an inclined surface (a ramp, a small hill, etc.) it seemed my legs had a mind of their own, and I was suddenly wearing lead weights. It was a chore to take the next step, yet I could walk up a flight of stairs with minimal effort. It was like the walking "switch" turned off. Even the smallest incline caught me off guard and a little argument with my mind and legs ensued. Through physical therapy, I learned that it wasn't just weak muscles and joints causing those inclines to be such a challenge but a proprioception/balance issue—one in which the physical therapist felt the stability of a cane could greatly benefit me.

I dared myself to run an errand with it (I was out of town where no one saw me.) Although I tripped myself a few times in the learning process (coordinating the oppo-site foot of cane-side took some getting used to), I quickly saw that I could walk up hills or on uneven surfaces with minimal effort, and with it, I no longer needed to seek a wall, a post, or something on which to keep me from swaying when standing still. The cane opened a new door for me that I didn't even realize had closed, and I gained a self-reliance I hadn't known for several years. After I started using it, a funny thing happened—*I found independence!*

First, I used it to get my mail. The uphill walk back from my mailbox was always a challenge.

Next, I used it when we met my son and his family at a cabin in the woods—there was only one way to get around without help as we walked to the river; once again my new but trusty cane brought me independence. I didn't need to rely on someone's arm, and I loved being able to get around on uneven terrain or hills without fear of falling. I still had to figure out how to manage the cane with weak hands. In addition, all this independence brought on more fatigue as I was now enjoying activities I hesitated to do on my own. Not long into using a cane outside the home, I became an advocate of its use for those whose balance has been affected by MS. You know what? Independence is pretty darned cool (and staying upright has its perks too!)

Not everyone experiences the same challenges and many may never need a cane at all, but take it from me, if you find yourself avoiding situations or social gatherings due to balance issues, do something about it!

For more information regarding measuring or pur-chasing the appropriate cane this link from Mayo Clinic is helpful: http://www.mayoclinic.org/healthy-lifestyle/healthy-aging/multimedia/canes/sls-20077060.

A healthy alternative to medications, physical/occupational, and speech therapy is worth considering. If you are anything like me, I'm not satisfied with "good enough." I want to try as many sensible alternatives as I can to help me maintain as much independence as possible.

Based on feedback from other people with RRMS or secondary progressive MS, Pilates, yoga, acupuncture, and specific therapeutic massage techniques from a licensed massage therapist can provide relieve of some symptoms and should be explored to see how they might benefit you.

Other Alternatives

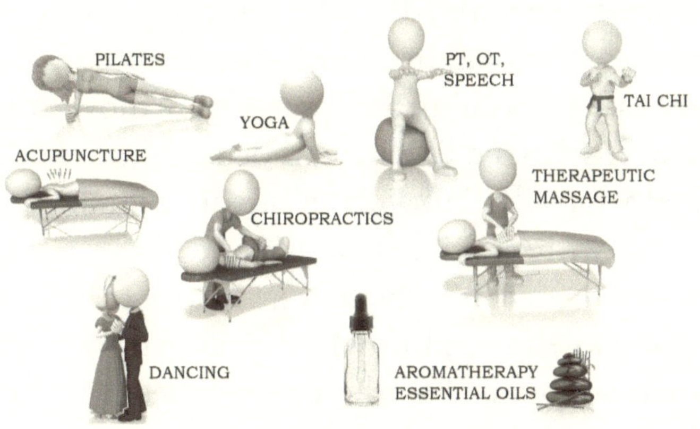

Yoga

Several years ago, I joined a beginner's yoga class at my local fitness center. With painful wrists, weak hands, and legs that kept going into spasms, I simply was not able to make that class work for me. Although it was for "beginners," the large class filled the crowded room with people who had been doing yoga for years, and the class moved too quickly for me to figure out how to adjust the movements to fit my limitations. I gave it an honest go but realized this particular class was not the right fit for me. I have read many testimonials of MS'ers who benefit from yoga. If taking a yoga class does not work for you, consider a beginner's yoga class on video or on-line. The National MS Society has a good reference article here:

https://nationalmssociety.org/NationalMSSociety/media/MSNationalFiles/Brochures/Yoga_A_Focus_on_Mild_Symptoms_Of_MS_Final.pdf

Pilates

A friend sent me information regarding the benefits of Pilates for people with MS, which included improvement in stability, core strengthening, improved posture and balance, increased flexibility and prevention and treatment of back pain. It sounded like I could benefit from Pilates, so I scheduled a consultation with an instructor trained to work with people with multiple sclerosis and began my training in a one-on-one environment. The instructor assessed my physical weaknesses and provided personal instruction on exercises that could offer the greatest benefit. I was surprised how much Pilates benefited me.

For example, that crazy "MS Hug" can be a real challenge for me as the muscles between my ribs feel like they are squeezing the very breath out of me. I told her about this sensation, and she showed me breathing techniques and exercises that addressed expanding the rib cage. Fortunately for me, Dennis is a licensed master massage therapist with over twenty years' experience. We have found a breathing/massage technique that greatly reduces the tightness in the rib-cage and brings much-needed relief when I'm experiencing it. That alone has made Pilates worth it! My plan is to continue Pilates as long as it continues to benefit me, and I strongly recommend this alternative for anyone with MS. Be sure you work with a trainer who understands multiple sclerosis.

Ballroom Dancing

After struggling with coordination and balance issues for several years, I was excited and surprised to read multiple articles about the positive neurological benefits of ballroom dancing…or any kind of dancing for that matter. Dennis and I had always loved dancing, but as life got busy and balance became a challenge, it was put on the back burner until recently. Dennis initiated ballroom dance lessons after reading scholarly articles about the benefits of this activity both physically and neurologically. Not only has it been a fun way to exercise our body and our mind, but hopefully, over time, it will improve my balance to some degree as well.

In an on-line article from Harvard Medical School Department of Neurobiology on Dancing and the Brain, the authors write "Scientists gave little thought to the neurological effects of dance until relatively recently, when researchers began to investigate the complex mental coordination that dance requires…" They go on to explain how "Music stimulates the brain's reward centers, while dance activates its sensory and motor circuits."[xxiv] If you have the resources and physical ability to do so, ballroom dance is another option to exercise your brain. You may not win a spot on Dancing with the Stars, but you may gain a little more control staying upright when taking a walk.

Tai Chi

I have found some excellent videos on the internet demonstrating Tai Chi for beginners and even if I have to sometimes modify the demonstration to fit my ability, I can do this Chinese martial art, (some would call it "a form of dance") in the privacy of my own living room, in my own timing, and with no one watching. Tai Chi is a gentle form of exercise and "mindfulness training" that most people with RRMS can do while standing (with or without assistance of a chair or wall.)

Tai Chi seems to have a positive affect on people with neurological disorders. For example, in a six-month study conducted in Germany, thirty-two people with MS were followed. About half participated in 90-minute, weekly Tai Chi program compared to the control group who did not participate. After six months, those who participated in the Tai Chi program showed not only significant improvement in balance and coordination, but they also had less depression and fatigue whereas the control group did not have these results.[xxv] If minor commitments toward improvement offer potential benefits, I want to take full advantage. I refuse to "sit back" and "let" MS win without giving it a good "fight."

Acupuncture

An age-old form of traditional Chinese medicine, acupuncture focuses on the fourteen pathways of energy flow throughout the body. Many of the comments I have read from people with MS state that acupuncture minimized or alleviated some of their MS-related pain, reduced the intensity of numbness and tingling, and greatly reduced incidences of spasticity and bladder problems. Some even stated that acupuncture seemed to lift their cloud of depression.

I understand that adjunct therapies can be cost prohibitive and few if any are covered by medical insurance, but if it is at all possible to give these alternatives a try, I strongly encourage you to do so.

MS Memory Toolbox

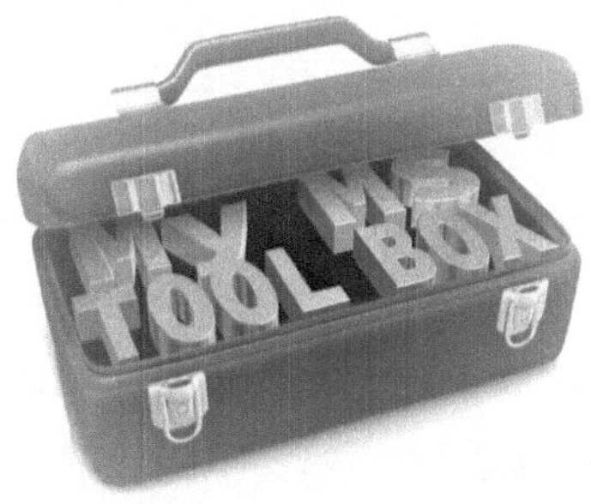

The great thing about technology is that it really can help us organize, remember, recall, record, and find our way to and from anywhere. Technology can help make life easier. Some tools you may have by your side right now. For example:

- Use your phone camera to snap pics of any visible symptoms you feel should be recorded. It's much easier to show your doctor a photo or video than to try to explain it, and it's amazing how they respond when they see it for themselves.

- As stated earlier, I have always had a bad sense of direction. However, when my "wires get crossed" and spatial awareness is inexplicably impaired, GPS is a tool sent straight from heaven.

- I use an online calendar on my phone/laptop and share it with Dennis so we can keep up with one another's appointments and activities that affect us both. I don't just use it to remember birthdays and anniversaries, but *all* commitments and appointments are in there as well. Modern technology lets us sync our calendar on our phone and laptop as well as share any or all of it with our partner.

- I use the "reminders" option in my calendar to pop up two days before, the day before, and two hours before an appointment. That may seem like "overkill" to some people, but for me, it's what I need.

- There are many free apps available which allow users to log vitals, prescriptions, photos or other medical information. Many allow users to share part or all the information with others or email portions of the information (i.e., my prescription list) as needed. Currently I use a free app called Care Zone (https://carezone.com/home), which allows me to share parts of my information with others I choose, log medications, use it for reminders and to log questions or concerns I need to share with my doctor at my next appointment.

- I use my oven and/or phone timer to remind me of everything. I wouldn't dream of cooking or doing anything that needs remembering without utilizing a timer to remind me. Yes, I am that forgetful, but I do at least remember to set the timer!

- The Memo app on my phone helps me control and remember tasks I need to complete, and I enter everything I need to do or buy on that app *as I think of it.* If I don't jot it down, I won't remember.

- Many grocery stores now offer online shopping, free delivery, and ready-to-pick-up options. What a great energy conservation tool this has been! If you run out of steam as quickly as I do, you will fully appreciate this option. I use the store app as my grocery list, and it's all there at the click of a button to pay and pick up.

- If you struggle with heat sensitivity, consider using a cooling vest, misting fan, or other tools that will help control heat exposure. As of this printing, both the Multiple Sclerosis Association of America (MSAA) and the Multiple Sclerosis Foundation (MSF) offer cooling vests or other cooling gear at no charge to eligible MS patients through the following websites: MSAA—https://mymsaa.org/msaa-help/cooling-products/ MSF—https://msfocus.org/Get-Help/MSF-Programs-Grants/Cooling-Program

- If hand strength or overall weakness is a problem for you, utilize tools that can make your life easier. (i.e. – electric can opener, jar openers, Velcro or slip-on vs. laced shoes, zippers vs. buttons…the list is endless.)
- Use grip bars to get in/out of the tub if slipping/falling is a concern. Use a shower chair and a detachable shower head if weakness or fatigue is an issue. There are adaptive devises available that address virtually every challenge with which you may be dealing.
- If traveling, consider using a wheelchair to avoid fatigue; obtain a gate pass if you need help through security. There is a *TSA Cares* hotline for travelers with disabilities or medical conditions and for individuals needing assistance. Their number is 855-787-2227.
- The list of useful tools available is endless and includes apps to improve memory, online support groups, yoga, and Pilates videos, etc.
- Remember tools are only useful if you use them.

Using Assistive Devices When Needed

If you've never needed an assistive device, fantastic! Many with MS are challenged to maintain balance or deal with symptoms that compromise their ability to get around without some type of assistance (someone's arm, a grocery cart, the walls and furniture of your house, etc.). Maybe you hold back because you are embarrassed; maybe you haven't had the final tumble that told you to stop resisting help; maybe you are afraid that if you use an assistive device of some sort you have "given up" and allowed MS "to win."

With the invisible symptoms of relapsing/remitting or secondary progressive MS, many are hesitant to use assistive devices because we know that others aren't in our bodies and can't know our arbitrary struggles. Maybe you are hesitant because you know that people tend to "judge" or you don't know how to explain that using wrist splints or a cane today or this week or this month or maybe only as you need it does appear inconsistent to those who don't understand the relapsing/remitting nature of the disease. The tendency is *not* to use assistive devices at all—but instead we endure the pain, hide the tools, and risk dropping things or even falling. Does that really make sense?

Rock that Cane

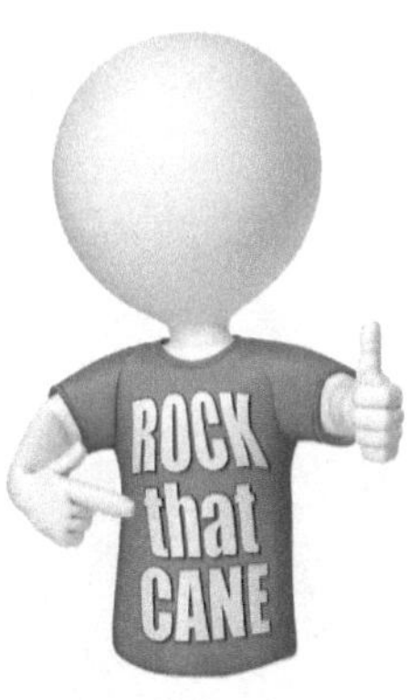

Although constant loss-of-balance moments have me "catching" myself (even when standing still), and although my physical therapist encouraged me to use a cane, I continued to do my best without one. Using the grocery cart, hubby's arm (or whatever) to help with stability, I just couldn't bring myself to use one. I knew I needed one, but it was just such a huge step for the Queen of Denial.

One day, in a text, I had mentioned the therapist's recommendation about using a cane to my daughter-in-law who was in nursing school at the time. She said, *"Embrace it! Rock that cane!"* That day, I ordered my first cane. But at the time, it was for "just in case." I confess, my thinking was: "I know myself enough to know that it will likely take a Humpty Dumpty moment before I resort to using a cane, but I do know these options are available should I need them …"

A few weeks later, I lost my balance in a clothing store at the mall. I fell backward in slow-motion into the clothing rack, breaking hangers and pulling clothing down as I grabbed at whatever I could in a failed attempt to stop the fall. Using a cane would have been *far* less obvious than tumbling fanny first to the floor and hitting my tail bone on the rack bar below while two young salesclerks ran over to me, shouting, "Oh no! Are you okay, ma'am?"

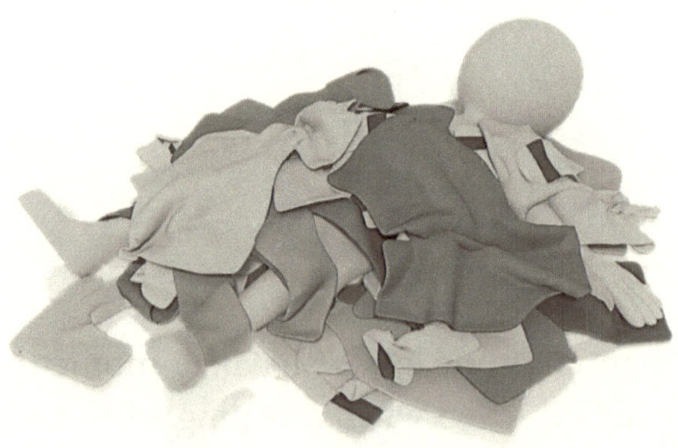

"Yes," I replied, "but my pride is a bit injured!"

MS symptoms can be ridiculously random. If you are reading this journal, you know there's nothing "fun" about using an assistive device whether for a short spell or for the long haul. Because RRMS can be so sporadic, there are times when using an assistive tool could benefit one greatly, and yet, for some people, not needed much or at all while in remission.

If your MS symptoms are more progressive, it is probably now a permanent tool; maybe you just use it when you're going out. Maybe you need a cane any time you're standing or when you first get up in the morning. When the simple task of standing still, walking, or going up or down inclines becomes a problem, it may be time to consider an assistive device.

I found that guidance from a physical therapist on how to select and use a cane was extremely beneficial. Keep in mind that choosing the wrong type of cane, the wrong height for you, or using a cane incorrectly can make matters worse.

If you don't need a cane at all—HURRAY for you! If you struggle but you're hesitant, don't wait for your Humpty Dumpty moment. I understand your hesitation and apprehension, but trust me when I say this, the independence I found when I had something to help me maintain balance has been well worth it!

Sticker Shock

After over twelve weeks of physical, occupational and speech therapy, I realized that the issues for which I was seeking help were not going to go away, and that, in fact, they would likely progress over time. I was encouraged by one of the therapists to consider a handicap parking sticker so I could park closer to my destination, help reduce fatigue, conserve energy and avoid falls. I looked around and saw people in wheelchairs or dealing with obvious handicaps and somehow just didn't allow myself permission to consider myself in this category as long as I was still able to stand upright.

However, excessive fatigue *always* had me driving home before completed errands, and following my uncontrolled backward tumble into the clothing rack at the mall (and an injured tailbone), I called my doctor. By then, he had received the therapists' assessment and post therapy notes and without hesitancy completed the form needed for the DMV to issue a "permanent disability" sticker. I could barely bring myself to hang it on my rearview mirror. "Is that *mine*?" I asked myself, "When did this happen?"

It happened over time. Little by little and relapse by relapse until my independence shrunk, my confidence to go out by myself faded, my sense of balance digressed, and I saw myself becoming Humpty Dumpty. Once again, I had to tell myself, "It's okay to get help and use new measures to live life to its fullest."

The first time I used the handicap tag, I had several errands to run, and I was exhausted from a long line of trips to and from stores. I had one last stop to make in the middle of town. I dared to place the handicap sticker on my rearview mirror and proceeded to find a handicap spot to "try on" my parking spot. But alas—there was not a handicap spot to be found *anywhere* in that small parking lot. I had to park a long way off to get that last errand done.

I chuckled at the thought that I had this sticker, but there was nowhere to park but the farthest end of the next store's parking lot.

So now, I *do* "rock that cane" and view it *not* as a "crutch" but as a tool to independence. I do use those handicap spaces when I feel I need it. It helps me conserve much needed energy to finish out my day without collapsing.

It doesn't mean we've "given up" or "given in" to use tools that keep us upright. It doesn't mean we've stopped fighting for ourselves or ceased to find other means to help us improve balance, maintain what we have or prolong losing more. It simply means we are doing the best we can to enjoy life to the fullest right now. In fact, I now have *several* canes to match my mood, my outfit or my situation. Before our vacation, Dennis even bought me an attachment that fit on the base of my cane to allow walking on a sandy beach! I guess I really have learned to "rock those canes!"

Using a Wheelchair or Scooter

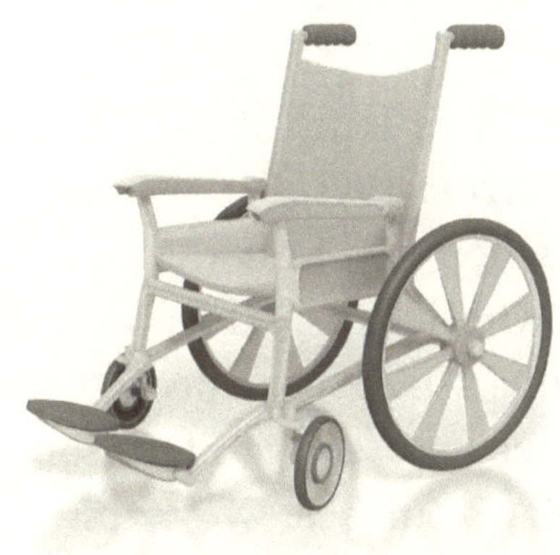

According to the National Multiple Sclerosis Society, people with MS experience a likely prognosis for a relatively normal life span. They may contend with some degree of disability, but most people with RRMS are not severely disabled. Many live with pain, discomfort, and inconvenience to some extent but have a great potential to living a healthy life. The big question for those with MS is, "Will I end up in a wheelchair?"

The degree of disability is dependent on the person, the stage of the disease or the amount/location of nerve damage. Two out of three people with relapsing-remitting or secondary progressive MS will be able to ambulate on their own throughout their lifetime. For some, a cane may be needed for balance or stability due to the faulty "messaging" in the brain that causes imbalance, instability with gait, or weakened muscles. Others may use a wheelchair from time to time during a physically exerting excursion (like the hike demanded at an airport or for other activities that can bring on excessive muscle fatigue.) The price one pays for exhaustion and muscle fatigue or falling can be far greater than the "awkwardness" of using a wheelchair in the first place.

In her article, "The Truth about MS and Wheelchairs," author Debbie Petrina says, "If you asked anyone 'what do you think of when you hear the term MS?' the answer usually includes 'wheelchairs.'" Her article states that "over their lifetime, only 20-25% of people with MS will end up needing a wheelchair (though far more will need a cane to help with balance/muscle weakness issues over time) because of fatigue, weakness, balance problems, or to assist with conserving energy."[xxvi]

While most people with MS may never *need* a wheelchair at all, it is recommended that patients consider its use if *not* using one puts you at risk of injury or unnecessary muscle fatigue. It's hard to explain to someone what it feels like to have muscle fatigue if they don't have MS, but the best example I can give is the feeling you would have if you walked up a set of endless stairs until you could no longer take another step—your muscles simply say, "Enough!" Pushing oneself to the point of muscle fatigue can result in *excruciating* muscle spasms that can last hours without relenting or spasticity that can last even longer.

If MS symptoms have progressed enough that muscle fatigue puts you at risk of falling, a wheelchair can be a *preventative* tool for you. Don't be ashamed or embarrassed to use one. You owe *no one* an explanation, and it doesn't mean that you have now "moved into it" for good. Many people with MS have learned that they can participate in outings they would not have enjoyed before simply by using a chair for as much or as little as needed.

Get to know yourself, your abilities and your disabilities, then *take heart*. Life is grand even if it means having to hold someone's arm, use a cane, or even "hitch a ride" in a chair to navigate more safely as the situation deems necessary.

Handling "Recall Misfires"

Most of us have experienced what we jokingly call "senior moments," "brain farts," or "I forgot what I was just saying." Misfires for anyone (with or without MS) can be caused by distraction, low blood sugar, aging, medication side effects, a stressful time in a person's life, or even having "too much on our plates." We all know what I'm talking about here.

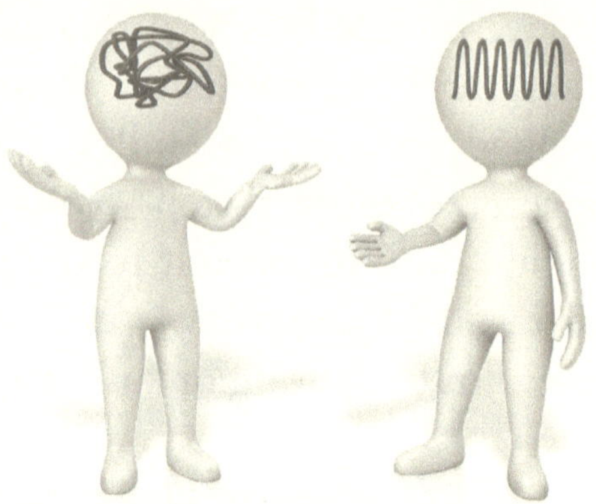

Cognitive malfunction is a common symptom with MS and affects more than two out of three MS patients, a result of the loss of myelin that surrounds the nerves of the central nervous system (CNS). Sclerosis is the culprit that incites disruption or interference in the transportation of information to the brain. It can cause cognitive "hiccups" such as information processing from the five senses, concentration issues, attention deficits, retention or retrieval of information from the "memory bank," the ability to prioritize or plan (executive functions), visual disturbances and/or the ability to find a word "at the tip of your tongue." People with MS may have minor or major problems with these functions. They may deal with cognitive issues occasionally or often, and they may experience difficulties with only a few or many of these cognitive functions depending on where the damage is located on the brain. It can be exasperating when recall misfire occurs in the middle of a conversation.

All Aboard … Tickets Please!

One of the ways I have dealt with recall misfires when out in public is to hand the person with whom I am chatting what I call my "MS Ticket." I created these several years ago to give me a "way out" of an embarrassing moment and to use these "misfire" moments as an opportunity to educate others about multiple sclerosis. I can go months without needing them or weeks when I keep them handy in my pocket or purse. I have had positive feedback from those with whom I've shared my "tickets."

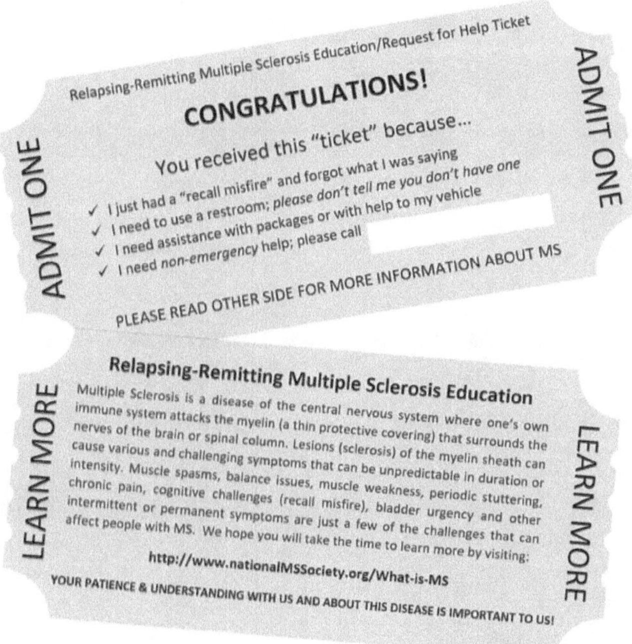

Whether you choose to use "tickets" or have your own creative way to deal with the symptoms of MS, the most important "take away" is that you not allow MS to dictate your life or allow you to "recluse" or "hide" when you're in relapse or dealing with symptoms. For more information on ordering your own "MS Tickets", contact JustATadDitzy@gmail.com

CHAPTER FOURTEEN

BE YOUR OWN ADVOCATE

I had to learn to fight for myself when it came to being heard by the medical community. My experiences as well as my "gut" told me many years ago that my underlying problem was not just "epilepsy," but rather the seizures were a symptom of something going on that had not yet been identified. If it had been up to the neurologists, I would probably still be on anticonvulsants today—twenty years later!

I had to repeat myself *countless times*, and like a broken record, I told every doctor I ever saw that the symptoms with which I was dealing had a beginning—a date in time when I knew that "something" had changed for me. I have been affected for *two decades* with the symptoms described in this journal, and for the most part, though only one doctor acted as though he didn't "believe" me, all others were caring and more "baffled" than disbelieving and understandably so.

This advice is for anyone with any disease: *Be your own advocate.* You know how you feel—and you know these symptoms are real. If your family physician, specialist or neurologist doesn't seem to care or listen—*run!* Find a doctor who cares.

I learned many years ago that I needed to look after myself and do my own homework. Thankfully, outstanding information, scholarly articles, and reputable MS specific educational websites are at our fingertips. When advocating for yourself, the most important message I can share is *don't give up*—find a doctor who takes you seriously. If you feel it would benefit you, consider joining an online or local support group that deals specifically with multiple sclerosis. They are often helpful in directing you to helpful, informative, free materials, online videos, educational pamphlets, brochures, and other resources.

You can find more information and connections to support groups through these and other sites:

- The Mayo Clinic: https://www.mayoclinic.org/diseases-conditions/multiple-sclerosis/diagnosis-treatment/drc- 20350274
- Medline Plus: https://medlineplus.gov/multiplesclerosis.html
- The US National Library of Medicine: https://www.ncbi.nlm.nih.gov/pubmedhealth/PMHT0024311/
- MS International Federation: https://www.msif.org/
- National MS Society: https://www.nationalmssociety.org/Resources-Support/Find-Support
- The Multiple Sclerosis Association of America https://mymsaa.org/

CHAPTER FIFTEEN

REDEFINING WHO YOU ARE

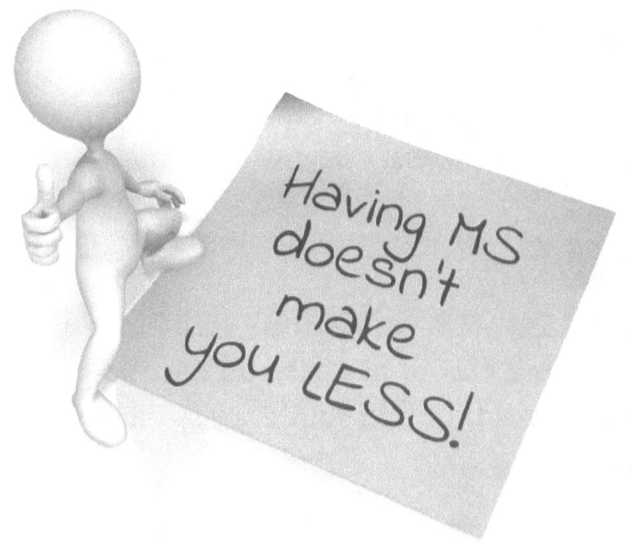

If you have fallen into the trap of becoming reclusive, hiding, or "faking it," take heart and remember this, *just because you have MS doesn't make you less!*

The first step is to educate yourself, understand your own disease so you can recognize symptoms and triggers, then educate those you love so they can know what it is you're dealing with. Personally, I don't care if strangers don't understand, but I do care that those I'm close to understand.

Don't believe the lies inside your head; stay positive and hang with people who are positive too.

Don't allow yourself to use self-deprecating language like "idiot" or "stupid" or "crazy." You are none of these, and it's not your fault that you have a disease that affects you physically, cognitively, and sometimes emotionally.

If you don't have a significant other that teams with you through life's goofy, unpredictable MS "adventures," consider checking out a support group or a church community group or contacting the National MS Society. Their toll-free number is 1-800-344-4867. http://www.nationalmssociety.org/Resources-Support/Find-Support/Edward-M-Dowd-Personal-Advocate-Program.

If you don't already know this, let me remind you—*you are loved by God!*

Psalm 139:1–18, a beautiful and inspirational poem written by King David, has been an encouragement to me for decades. I read it often to lift my spirit and to keep me grounded.

O LORD, You have searched me and known *me*.
You know when I sit down and when I rise up;
You understand my thought from afar.
You scrutinize my path and my lying down,
And are intimately acquainted with all my ways.
Even before there is a word on my tongue,
Behold, O LORD, YOU KNOW IT ALL.
You have enclosed me behind and before,
And laid Your hand upon me.
Such knowledge is too wonderful for me;
It is *too* high, I cannot attain to it.
Where can I go from Your Spirit?
Or where can I flee from Your presence?
If I ascend to heaven, You are there;
If I make my bed in Sheol, behold, You are there.
If I take the wings of the dawn,
If I dwell in the remotest part of the sea,
Even there Your hand will lead me,
And Your right hand will lay hold of me.
If I say, "Surely the darkness will overwhelm me,
And the light around me will be night,"
Even the darkness is not dark to You,
And the night is as bright as the day.
Darkness and light are alike *to You*.
For You formed my inward parts;
You wove me in my mother's womb.
I will give thanks to You, for I am fearfully
and wonderfully made;
Wonderful are Your works,
And my soul knows it very well.

My frame was not hidden from You,
When I was made in secret,
And skillfully wrought in the depths of the earth;
Your eyes have seen my unformed substance;
And in Your book were all written the days
that were ordained *for me*,
When as yet there was not one of them.
How precious also are Your thoughts to me,
O God!
How vast is the sum of them!
If I should count them, they would outnumber the sand.
When I awake, I am still with You.
(Psalm 139:1–18, NASB)

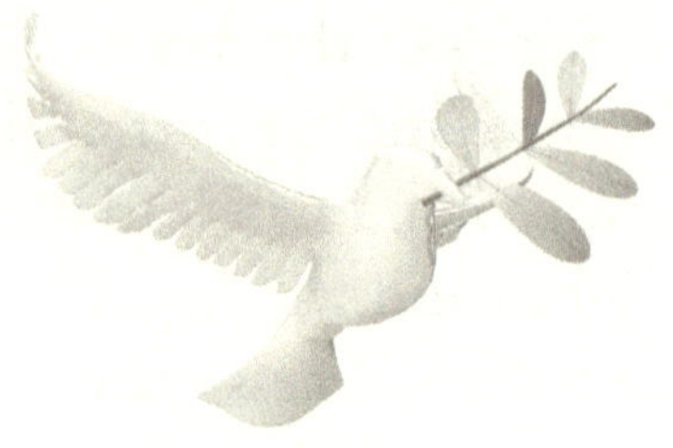

CHAPTER SIXTEEN

CONCLUSION

It is my goal that you have been enlightened, entertained, and educated in the process of reading this book and that you have claimed for yourself the fullest life possible without letting the effects of multiple sclerosis (or any disease) dictate your joy.

While I don't consider myself "a professional writer," I do see myself as an ordinary person who has been blessed greatly with extraordinary people in my life. This book began as my awkward attempt to deal with a disease I knew nothing about but had affected me for nearly fifteen years before diagnosis. It became a tool through which I was able to recognize how being undiagnosed for so long had affected me and how the same experiences also challenged me to grow in my faith and as an individual.

Researching and writing became a remarkable tool in helping me understand my own journey, in recognizing how MS had affected me in so many ways, in giving me ideas and resources for dealing with MS in the most effective way and in providing me the challenge to start anew. I trust that my loved ones have a better understanding of this disease, and I pray this book helps you and those you love to better understand and navigate your way more effectively through the complex MS maze.

Yes, MS sucks. But so does aging and cancer and arthrogryposis and rheumatoid arthritis and heart disease and diabetes and mental illness and kidney disease and liver failure and fibromyalgia and stroke and lung disease and any other disease with which this world and the people in it are plagued.

While we live in a broken world that doesn't discriminate between young or old or rich or poor or male or female when it comes to illnesses, we all have access to a great and mighty God who promises better things to come and is here to hold each of our hands through it all—if we would just let Him.

I REFUSE to allow
MULTIPLE SCLEROSIS
to define me.
I am so much more than just
"someone with MS."
I am me.
A wife. A lover. A neat freak. A mother.
A laugher. A joker. A bubble bath soaker.
A grandma. A writer. A neighbor. A fighter.
A dog lover, poet, if it's torn - I sew it.
A backyard gardener (addicted to books),
A friend. A foodie. A not-so-great cook.
At times I may think, "Good Lord, I'm a mess!"
Then I remember –
I'm a beloved child of GOD – *and nothing less!*

If you have benefited from the information and experiences expressed in this book, I would love to hear from you! Send me an email: JustATadDitzy@gmail.com

THANKS, CREDITS, ENDNOTES

Extra Special Thanks

To my husband and dearest friend on planet earth: Dennis, your unending encouragement, partnership of faith, unconditional love, and fun-loving humor have made my life a breeze and a blessing! *I appreciate you deeply.*

To my children: Brandon, Derek, April, and your beloved spouses who I love like my own children, *I could never say "thank you" enough for your ongoing encouragement and genuine support. I love each of you endlessly!*

To my beloved grandchildren: Boston, Caden, Riley, Emily, Eli, Kate, Kasie, and "Bug," *YOU are the shining lights of my day—I can't imagine this world without you in it!*

To my siblings: Paul, Emile, Jeannine, Ellen, Ray, and Angie and each of your beloved spouses: I *am deeply thankful that you are not only my beloved siblings, but also my dearest friends and closest prayer warriors.*

To Maryse and Dan: You have traveled this road far deeper and far longer than I. Thank you for your courage and for the example you have set in finding joy in every situation. *You are my heroes!*

To my life-long friends: Sally and Wayne Gustafson, John "Jay" Baseler, and Joan Hutchins, you have been a part of my life for decades (and decades!) *I'm a better person for sharing it with you.*

To Mike Sisco (BSc Exercise and Sports Sciences) - Thank you for showing me that I can do WAY more than I thought I could! You are topnotch! *In just a short time, I've learned SO MUCH working with you – it is life changing!*

To Cindy and Eric Stark – Thank you for "taking a chance" on me; God used you to bless and to change the direction of our lives. *We're thankful that you listened to Him!*

Credits

Thank you to www.PresenterMedia.com for permission to use the images for this book. For a subscription to Presenter Media, visit their website.

Endnotes

[i] Donati, Donatella and Jacobson, Seven. (2002 ASM Press, Bookshelf ID: NBK2494) Polymicrobial Diseases Chapter 6 Viruses and Multiple Sclerosis, under the paragraph "Neuropathology" Retrieved February 8, 2017 from https://www.ncbi.nlm.nih.gov/books/NBK2494/.

[ii] Donati, Donatella and Jacobson, Seven. (2002 ASM Press, Bookshelf ID: NBK2494) Polymicrobial Diseases Chapter 6 Viruses and Multiple Sclerosis, under the paragraph "Viruses Associated with MS". Retrieved February 8, 2017 from https://www.ncbi.nlm.nih.gov/books/NBK2494/.

[iii] Keegan, Mark MD. Multiple Sclerosis: Can It Cause Seizures: Is there any connection between multiple sclerosis and epilepsy? (2015 May) Retrieved December 27, 2016 from http://www.mayoclinic.org/diseases-conditions/multiple-sclerosis/expert-answers/multiple-sclerosis/faq-20058138.

iv What Causes MS? Infectious Factors, accessed February 8, 2017 http://www.nationalmssociety.org/What-is-MS/What-Causes-MS.

v Multiple Sclerosis Association of America: Possible Causes of Multiple Sclerosis, accessed February 26, 2017 http a first trigger of disease.://mymsaa.org/ms-information/overview/possible-causes/.

vi Mayo Clinic Staff. Diseases that Cause Bell's Palsy—Causes. Retrieved February 26, 2017 from http://www.mayoclinic.org/diseases-conditions/bells-palsy/basics/causes/con-20020529.

vii Arch Neurol. (2007) Multiple Sclerosis After Infectious Mononucleosis. Retrieved May 22, 2017 from https://www.ncbi.nlm.nih.gov/pubmed/17210811.

viii What is an immune-mediated disease? Overview. Retrieved December 24, 2017 https://www.nationalmssociety.org/What-is-MS/Definition-of-MS/Immune-mediated-disease.

ix Definition of MS, Retrieved December 24, 2017 https://www.nationalmssociety.org/What-is-MS/Definition-of-MS.

x Relapsing/Remitting MS (RRMS); Overview, Retrieved December 2, 2017 https://www.nationalmssociety.org/What-is-MS/Types-of-MS/Relapsing-remitting-MS.

xi Neurology and Neurosurgery; Multiple Sclerosis (MS), "Secondary Progressive Multiple Sclerosis (MS)" Retrieved January 11, 2018 from https://www.hopkinsmedicine.org/neurology_neurosurgery/centers_clinics/multiple_sclerosis/conditions/index.html.

xii Kuchinscas, Susan (2011). Why Do You Always Get Lost? Retrieved January 10, 2017 from http://www.webmd.com/brain/features/why-do-you-always-get-lost#1.

xiii Common Multiple Sclerosis-Related Cognitive Problems, Visual Perceptual Skills. Retrieved December 12, 2017 from http://www.dummies.com/health/common-multiple-sclerosis-related-cognitive-problems/.

xiv MS and Walking, Balance, & Coordination Problems, Retrieved November 5, 2017 https://multiplesclerosis.net/living-with-ms/ms-and-walking-balance-coordination-problems/.

xv Medical Marijuana (Cannabis). Guideline from American Academy of Neurology (March 24, 2014) Retrieved December 14, 2017 from https://www.nationalmssociety.org/Treating-MS/Complementary-Alternative-Medicines/Marijuana.

xvi Paull, Hannah (July 26, 2017). 5 Myths About Cannabis and MS, Retrieved December 14, 2017 from https://www.mssociety.org.uk/get-involved/campaigns/campaigns-blog/2017/07/5-myths-about-cannabis-and-ms.

xvii Momentum Magazine, the Magazine of the National MS Society entitled Invisible Symptoms in MS: how to help others "see" Your Symptoms—and How They Affect You; Counteracting Judgments Retrieved February 8, 2017 from http://www.momentummagazineonline.com/invisible-symptoms-ms/.

xviii Rolak, Loren MD. Multiple Sclerosis: It's Not the Disease You Thought It Was (January 2003) Retrieved December 16, 2016 from https://www.ncbi.nlm.nih.gov/pmc/articles/PMC1069023/.

xix MAGNETIC RESONANCE IMAGING (MRI) Uses in MS. Retrieved January 10, 2017 from http://www.nationalmssociety.org/Symptoms-Diagnosis/Diagnosing-Tools/MRI.

xx Wahls, Terry MD, The Wahls Protocol A Radical New Way to Treat All Chronic Autoimmune Conditions Using Paleo

Principles (Page 49). Published by The Penguin Group (USA) 2014. New York

xxi American Medical Association. State Law Chart: Naturopath Licensure and Scope of Practice Retrieved June 10, 2018 from https://www.ama-assn.org/sites/default/files/media-browser/specialty%20group/arc/ama-chart-naturopath-scope-practice-2017.pdf

xxii Multiple Sclerosis Association of America. S.E.A.R.C.H.™ for Treatment Options. What is S.E.A.R.C.H.™? Retrieved June 5, 2018 from https://mymsaa.org/ms-information/search/

xxiii Watson, Stephanie, (2015, December) How to Treat and Prevent an MS Flare-Up Retrieved December 21, 2016 from http://www.webmd.com/multiple-sclerosis/features/flare-ups#1.

xxiv Harvard Medical School. Department of Neurobiology. The Harvard Mahoney Neuroscience Institute Letter written by Scott Edwards. Retrieved June 13, 2018 from http://neuro.hms.harvard.edu/harvard-mahoney-neuroscience-institue/brain-newsletter/and-brain-series/dancing-and-brain

xxv Burschka, Keune, Hofstadt-van Oy, Oschmann, Kuhn. BMC Neurology, 2014. Mindfulness-based Interventions in Multiple Sclerosis: Beneficial Effects of Tai Chi on Balance, Coordination, Fatigue, and Depression. Retrieved June 13, 2018 from https://bmcneurol.biomedcentral.com/articles/10.1186/s12883-014-0165-4

xxvi Petrin, Debbie (2014, September) Managing MS—The Truth About MS and Wheelchairs, Retrieved September 5, 2017 from http://blog.debbiems.com/?p=370.

ABOUT THE AUTHOR

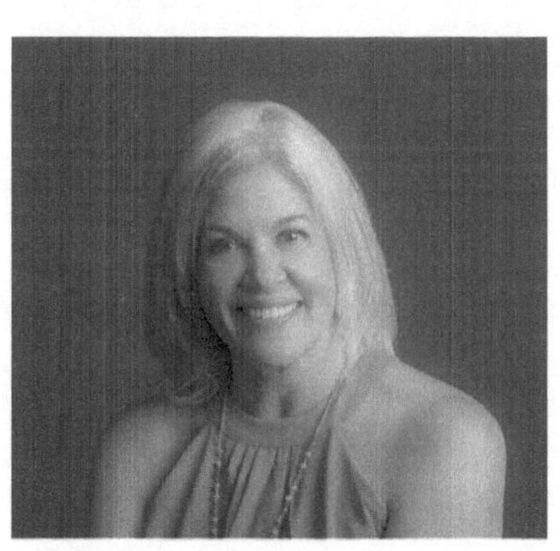

The sixth born of seven siblings, Jeanne was born in Woonsocket, Rhode Island, where she met and married her high school sweetheart, Dennis Champagne. During their "hippy phase," they traveled the country with their two young sons and eventually settled in Fayetteville, AR, in 1977. The following year, both Jeanne and Dennis became Christians, and their lives together were altered and bonded as never before. By 1983, they added to their family through adoption, and set out on life's journey as Christians, parents, and partners in life.

A poet and songwriter, Jeanne chronicled her life through journals, poetry, and music. Having written over four hundred songs, multiple musical dramas, poems, and written works, she also wrote, sang, and played in a Christian band for nearly twenty years, and with the band, recorded multiple inspiring albums.

Following a severe bout with the flu in 1997 an aspect of Jeanne's life changed as seizures and a multitude of symptoms plagued her intermittently for nearly fifteen years.

Her lighthearted, informative storytelling makes this book an easy read about her journey to diagnosis with relapsing-remitting multiple sclerosis, the challenges of being undiagnosed for so long, and her encouragement to others for claiming a full and happy life. Describing her life as "far too magnificent to get stuck along the way", Jeanne shares her story so that others can not only understand a little more about RRMS but also claim the freedom God gave us to claim the best possible life in spite of it.